TABLE OF CONTENTS

TABLE OF CONTENTS

Assessment of Risk in the Term Newborn

Susan Bakewell-Sachs, PhD, CRNP, RN, CS
Valerie D. Shaw, MS, RN
Amy L. Tashman, MSN, RNC

Editor
Lynn G. Wellman, MS, RNC
Nurse Educator
March of Dimes Birth Defects Foundation
White Plains, New York

Consulting Editor
Margaret Comerford Freda, EdD, RN, CHES, FAAN
Associate Professor
Department of Obstetrics, Gynecology, and Women's Health
Albert Einstein College of Medicine
Montefiore Medical Center
Bronx, New York

Library of Congress Cataloging-in-Publication Data

Bakewell-Sachs, Susan.

Assessment of risk in the term newborn / Susan Bakewell-Sachs. Valerie D. Shaw, Amy L. Tashman : editor, Lynn G. Wellman : consulting editor, Margaret Comerford Freda.

p. cm.

Includes bibliographical references.

ISBN 0-86525-074-X

1. Infants (Newborn)—Health risk assessment—Programmed instruction. 2. Pediatric nursing—Programmed instruction. 3. Infants (Newborn—Diseases—Diagnosis—Programmed instruction. I. Shaw, Valerie D. (Valerie Delores) II. Tashman, Amy L. III. Wellman, Lynn G. IV. March of Dimes Birth Defects Foundation V. Title.

[DNLM: 1. Neonatal Nursing—programmed instruction. 2. Nursing Assessment—programmed instruction. 3. Infant, Newborn. 4. Risk Factors. WY 18.2 B168a 1997]
RJ255.6.H4B35 1997
618.92'01—dc21
DNLM/DLC   97-8218
for Library of Congress   CIP

Published by:
Education Services
March of Dimes Birth Defects Foundation

Editor
Lynn G. Wellman, MS, RNC

Project Manager
Dorothy Drumgoole, MA

The mission of the March of Dimes Birth Defects Foundation is to improve the health of babies by preventing birth defects and infant mortality. To achieve this end, the Foundation funds programs of community service, advocacy, research and education. Part of our educational objective includes producing high-quality, low-cost educational resources for health care providers including March of Dimes nursing modules; assessment tools designed to enhance the skills of professionals who work with pregnant women; and videos and brochures to help providers communicate key reproductive health messages to clients.

Some of our publications may, on occasion, contain controversial views. All such statements and opinions are the sole responsibility of the authors, and do not reflect an endorsement by the March of Dimes Birth Defects Foundation or the editors, unless expressly stated.

To order additional copies of this or any other March of Dimes nursing module, or to request a free March of Dimes professional education catalog, please contact:

March of Dimes Fulfillment Center
P.O. Box 1657
Wilkes-Barre, PA 18703
Phone: 800-367-6630
Fax: 717-825-1987

For further information on March of Dimes nursing modules, write or call:

Education Services
March of Dimes Birth Defects Foundation
1275 Mamaroneck Avenue
White Plains, NY 10605
914-997-4456
E-mail: profedu@modimes.org

TABLE OF CONTENTS

Figures and Tables

Editor's Acknowledgements

Special thanks to authors **Susan Bakewell-Sachs, PhD, CRNP, RN, CS; Valerie D. Shaw, MS, RN**; and **Amy L. Tashman, MSN, RNC,** for making their knowledge available to many nurses and health care providers through the publication of this module.

We also gratefully acknowledge the following reviewer who so generously shared her expertise:

Susan T. Blackburn, PhD, RN, FAAN, Professor, Family and Child Nursing, University of Washington School of Nursing, Seattle, Washington.

Preface

March of Dimes nursing modules provide quality continuing education for nurses who deliver services to mothers and infants in a variety of health care settings. Recent years have seen dramatic changes in the world. All segments of society have been affected, altering our patterns of thinking, our actions, and reactions. Technological advances have changed medical and nursing practice. Changing demographics have created new opportunities for providers to serve childbearing families of diverse cultural backgrounds.

The March of Dimes recognizes the need to incorporate new, practical information and theoretical knowledge into nursing practice. To meet this challenge and promote excellent care for mothers and infants, the March of Dimes regularly convenes its Nurse Advisory Council to evaluate the nursing modules, to determine their direction, and to recommend development of new titles addressing vital issues confronting nurses today.

General Information

Nursing modules are self-directed learning monographs written by expert nurses for nursing professionals who provide prenatal or perinatal care. Each module addresses a specific topic and provides practical clinical information. Topics range from preconception to the neonatal period and cover changes that occur during the transition from intrauterine to extrauterine life; care of the pregnant woman and her fetus; the labor and delivery period; care of the postpartum client and her neonate; and current and future critical perinatal health problems. Each module provides background information and caregiving standards to meet these issues and addresses assessment of risk, stabilization of the client, and emergency care.

Nursing modules do not supplant didactic educational and clinical experiences for the topics covered. Rather, they are designed to provide registered nurses with information to enhance their existing baseline skills. Differential experiences of the learner may require various levels of guidance to apply the materials to practice; for modules that deal with advanced practice topics, clinical application may initially require close supervision.

Module Format

Each nursing module includes several interrelated components and sections. *Cognitive Objectives* are rooted in the factual nature of each module. *Expected Practice Outcomes* stem from the clinical implications of these facts. *Key Concepts* are included to facilitate identification of major points. The *Pre/Postinstructional Measurement* is designed to measure learner knowledge of the topic before and after module completion. *Clinical Application* emphasizes and provides reinforcement for clinical aspects of the material and allows transfer and implementation by the learner in a specific clinical setting. *Group Discussion Items* provide additional input from other learners and allow further exploration of cognitive and clinical objectives. *Supplementary Materials* provide annotated descriptions of multimedia resources to further enhance the module topic.

Getting the Most from the Module

To make the best use of a nursing module, learners should first read the *Cognitive Objectives, Expected Practice Outcomes,* and *Key Concepts* and then answer and correct the *Pre/Postinstructional Measurement.* They should then read the module text and proceed to the *Clinical Application.* If the module is being used in a group setting, the facilitator will arrange a meeting to discuss the *Clinical Application* and *Group Discussion Items.* As needed, learners should review the *References* and *Supplementary Materials* to reinforce the module content and its utilization in clinical practice.

Evaluation

An evaluation is printed on colored paper and inserted in the module. Please remove and complete the evaluation, fold and staple it to reveal the postage-paid portion, and post it in a U.S. mailbox. (Note: Group study participants may give the completed evaluation to their facilitator following the study session. Independent study takers may submit the completed evaluation, along with the test and required fee, directly to the March of Dimes. See the *Independent Study Application* for specific instructions.) Ongoing analysis of evaluations provides valuable data that enables the March of Dimes to offer the best possible continuing education for nurses.

Continuing Education Credit

This Educational Design II is presented by the March of Dimes Birth Defects Foundation, which has been approved as a provider of continuing education by the New York State Nurses Association's Council on Continuing Education, which is accredited by the American Nurses' Credentialing Center's Commission on Accreditation. **It has been assigned code MRCHDIMES-PRV-97-9736 and has been approved for 5.0 contact hours for registered nurses.** The March of Dimes is also approved as a continuing education provider by the State of California Board of Registered Nursing, Provider #CEP-11444.

To qualify for continuing education credit, participants must successfully complete the nursing module via independent study (requires a $35 processing fee) or facilitated group study as part of a hospital or other agency program, workshop, grand rounds, or conference.

Independent Study

To receive continuing education credit for independent study, each participant must:
1. Be a registered nurse or certified nurse-midwife
2. Purchase ($15) and read the module
3. Complete the *Independent Study Application* located at the back of the module
4. Complete the module evaluation (self-mailer)
5. Submit the completed *Independent Study Application* along with the module evaluation and a $35 check made payable to March of Dimes to: March of Dimes Nursing Modules, 1275 Mamaroneck Avenue, White Plains, NY 10605

The March of Dimes will notify participants of test results within six weeks of receiving the test. Participants with scores of 70% or higher will receive a certificate of completion; participants with scores less than 70% will be offered a second attempt to pass the test.

Facilitated Group Study

(Workshop/Grand Rounds/Conference)
A facilitated group study requires facilitation by a qualified registered nurse. A facilitated group study may occur as an inservice education program, a workshop or nursing grand rounds, or may be a portion of a larger conference or educational meeting. To receive continuing education credit for facilitated group study, each participant must:
1. Be a registered nurse or certified nurse-midwife
2. Purchase ($15) and read the module prior to the facilitated group study
3. Participate in the facilitated group study
4. Provide first and last name, address, and social security number

The facilitator must:

1. Be a registered nurse
2. Arrange time and location for the group study (minimum 60 minutes)
3. Facilitate discussion on the content of the module as well as the *Clinical Application and Group Discussion Items*
4. Submit a written request for certificates of completion on official agency/hospital/facility letterhead to:
   March of Dimes Nursing Modules, 1275 Mamaroneck Avenue, White Plains, NY 10605. The request must include the following:
   • Module title
   • Date, time, and location of facilitated group study
   • Participant list with first and last names, addresses, and social security numbers (A sign-in sheet is provided at the end of this section.)
   • Participant evaluations (tear-out self-mailer)

The host agency/hospital/facility must maintain the following for five years following completion of the activity:
• A copy of the participant list with first and last names, addresses, and social security numbers
• A copy of the module
• Curriculum vitae of the facilitator
• Summary of participant evaluations

Note: If a nursing module is used as part of a larger conference activity that is approved for continuing education credit and continuing education credit is to be awarded for a facilitated group study on the nursing module, use the following formula to calculate the appropriate amount of credit: The number of contact hours approved for the conference minus the number of contact hours counted for the facilitated group study time plus the number of contact hours approved for the module. See the following chart for an example:

Description	Credits
Full-day conference approved for seven contact hours	7.0
Minus one conference hour for the facilitated group study using the *Assessment of Risk in the Term Newborn* module	-1.0
Plus six hours approved for the facilitated group study on the *Assessment of Risk in the Term Newborn* module	+ 5.0
Equals the total number of contact hours awarded for the conference plus the facilitated group study	**= 11.0**

About This Module

The purpose of the *Assessment of Risk in the Term Newborn* module is to provide the perinatal nurse with essential information to assess the newborn's physiologic adaptation to extrauterine life and to assess for infectious or metabolic disorders. Gestational age assessment, physical assessment and newborn behavior patterns are discussed. Nursing management during the early newborn period is outlined, including identification of risk factors, assessment, monitoring and intervention during hospitalization and postdischarge followup.

March of Dimes

of Dimes

Saving babies, together

Assessment of Risk in the Term Newborn

Facilitated Group Study Participant Roster

Facilitator _____ **Date** _____

Location _____

*This sign-in sheet **may** be used to record participation in the facilitated group study. Facilitators should submit a participant roster to the March of Dimes following completion of the facilitated group study activity. **PLEASE PRINT LEGIBLY.***

	Last Name	First Name	Credentials	Mailing Address	Social Security #
1					
2					
3					
4					
5					
6					
7					
8					
9					
10					
11					
12					
13					
14					
15					
16					
17					
18					
19					
20					

Susan Bakewell-Sachs

BSN, University of Pittsburgh, Pittsburgh, Pennsylvania

MSN, University of Pennsylvania, Philadelphia, Pennsylvania

PhD, University of Pennsylvania, Philadelphia, Pennsylvania

PNP, University of Pennsylvania, Philadelphia, Pennsylvania

Susan Bakewell-Sachs is presently the coordinator of the Family Nurse Practitioner Program at The College of New Jersey, Ewing, New Jersey. Her clinical background includes neonatal intensive care, home follow-up care of high-risk infants and their families, and primary care of high-risk infants. Dr. Bakewell-Sachs practices one day per week in the high-risk clinic in the primary care center at the Children's Hospital of Philadelphia. Her primary research interest focuses on discharge management and long-term outcomes of preterm infants and their families.

Dr. Bakewell-Sachs is a member of the March of Dimes National Nurse Advisory Council, the Association of Women's Health, Obstetric and Neonatal Nurses, the National Association of Neonatal Nurses and Sigma Pheta Tau. She is certified as a pediatric nurse practitioner by the American Nurses' Credentialing Center.

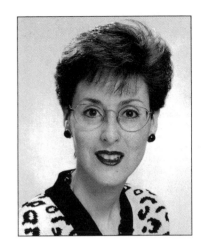

Valerie Shaw

BS, Rutgers University College of Nursing, Newark, New Jersey

MS, Rutgers University College of Nursing, Newark, New Jersey

Valerie Delores Shaw is the Nurse Manager of the Special Care Nurseries at the University of Pennsylvania Medical Center, Philadelphia, Pennsylvania.

She currently is certified as a Clinical Nurse Specialist in New Jersey. For the past eight years, Ms. Shaw has served as co-adjunct faculty in Maternal Child Health at Rutgers University School of Nursing. She is co-author of two chapters in an obstetric text and is presently writing additional articles for publication.

Ms. Shaw is a member of the National Association of Neonatal Nurses, the Delaware Valley Association of Neonatal Nurses, and Sigma Theta Tau.

Ms. Shaw is currently pursuing her doctorate in nursing at the University of Maryland.

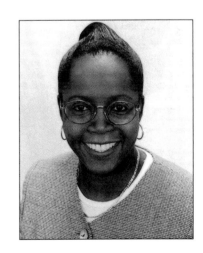

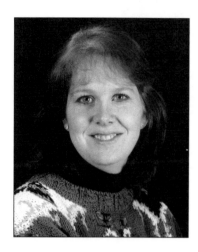

Amy L. Tashman, MSN, RNC

BSN, University of Pennsylvania School of Nursing, Philadelphia, Pennsylvania

MSN, University of Pennsylvania School of Nursing, Philadelphia, Pennsylvania

Amy Tashman is the Assistant Nurse Manager of the Special Care Nurseries at the University of Pennsylvania Medical Center, Philadelphia, Pennsylvania.

She currently is certified in Neonatal Intensive Care Nursing by the National Certification Corporation, and serves as a Neonatal Resuscitation Program Regional Trainer for the American Heart Association/American Academy of Pediatrics. She has also served as clinical faculty for undergraduate nursing students in Obstetric and Neonatal Nursing at the University of Pennsylvania School of Nursing.

Mrs. Tashman is a member of the National Association of Neonatal Nurses, the Delaware Valley Association of Neonatal Nurses, and the Association of Women's Health, Obstetric, and Neonatal Nurses.

Upon completion of this module, the learner will be able to:

1. Differentiate risk assessment findings between preterm, term and post-term gestations.

2. List the five components of the Apgar score.

3. Describe the four methods of heat loss in the newborn, and identify nursing management strategies to prevent cold stress in the nursery and delivery room.

4. Discuss methods of prevention and/or treatment for various perinatal infections.

5. Discuss newborns at risk for polycythemia and describe management criteria.

6. Discuss newborn behavioral states during the transition to extrauterine life, based on Brazelton's Neonatal Behavioral Assessment Scale.

7. Discuss metabolic screening tools and the disorders they are designed to detect.

8. Discuss the risk factors, symptoms and management of hypoglycemia and hyperglycemia.

9. Discuss the process of bilirubin metabolism, and identify the risk factors, symptoms and management of physiologic jaundice and non-physiologic jaundice.

The learner who meets the objectives and understands the key concepts for this module can be expected to:

1. Assign an appropriate Apgar score to a newborn infant.

2. Determine appropriate gestational age and classify as SGA, AGA or LGA, based on physical and neurological assessment.

3. Appropriately apply thermoregulation concepts in the neonatal period.

4. Monitor the newborn for signs/symptoms of perinatal infection.

5. Correctly obtain specimen(s) for newborn metabolic screening.

6. Delineate the nurse's role in the care of an infant with hypoglycemia and hyperglycemia.

7. Provide appropriate stabilization and eliminate factors that predispose the newborn to becoming hypoglycemic.

8. Distinguish between breast-milk jaundice and jaundice associated with breastfeeding.

9. Manage symptoms that are associated with physiologic and non-physiologic jaundice.

10. Appropriately manage the infant on phototherapy.

11. Assess the term newborn for risk of polycythemia.

The material in this module will help the learner understand the following concepts:

1. The Apgar score is indicative of the need for resuscitation, but not the degree of asphyxia.

2. Symptoms of hypoglycemia are frequently absent despite extremely low blood glucose levels.

3. Hyperglycemia is more prevalent in preterm and small-for-gestational-age newborns.

4. Heat loss in the newborn can occur through four mechanisms: conduction, convection, radiation and evaporation.

5. Inappropriate management of cold stress and heat stress in neonates has been associated with metabolic complications such as hypoglycemia, increased oxygen consumption, increased lactic acid production, increased metabolic acidosis and death.

6. Gestational age is the most predictive criterion for survival of the newborn infant.

7. Newborns follow a predictable set of behaviors as they transition to extrauterine life.

8. The best method of treatment for neonatal viral and bacterial infections is prevention.

9. Treatment of polycythemia is somewhat controversial, and is usually not provided unless symptoms are present.

10. Infants with extreme hyperbilirubinemia are at risk for developing bilirubin encephalopathy and kernicterus.

11. Therapeutic management of the newborn with hyperbilirubinemia is based on clinical judgment, history, course and clinical findings.

Instructions: Circle the BEST response for each question.

1. Which is not an immediate goal of transition to extrauterine life?

   A. Establishment of adequate respirations

   B. Effective thermoregulation

   C. Determination of gestational age

   D. Maintenance of euglycemia

2. Which terminology is associated with an infant whose birthweight is at the 50th percentile when gestational age is considered:

   A. Small for gestational age

   B. Appropriate for gestational age

   C. Preterm

   D. Intrauterine growth restricted

3. What is the most common clinical finding in newborns infected with Neisseria gonorrhoeae?

   A. Hepatitis

   B. Rhinitis

   C. "Blueberry muffin" rash

   D. Ophthalmia neonatorum (conjunctivitis)

4. What is a common clinical finding in newborns infected with congenital syphilis?

   A. Hepatitis

   B. Bullous vesicular eruptions

   C. "Blueberry muffin" rash

   D. Ophthalmia neonatorum (conjunctivitis)

5. Hypoglycemia is defined as symptoms occurring in conjunction with a blood glucose level of less than:

   A. 40 mg/dl

   B. 50 mg/dl

   C. 65 mg/dl

   D. 80 mg/dl

6. The stored form of glucose is:

   A. Glycerol

   B. Glycogen

   C. Pyruvate

   D. Insulin

7. Infants of diabetic mothers show symptoms of tremors, apnea, cyanosis and poor sucking reflex because of:

   A. Depression of the islets of langerhans

   B. Hypoglycemia

   C. CNS edema

   D. Hyperglycemia

8. Which of the following is a potential complication of hyperglycemia?

   A. Osmotic diuresis

   B. Hyperosmolarity

   C. Hyperbilirubinemia

   D. Rebound hypoglycemia

9. Hyperbilirubinemia in the term neonate is defined as a serum bilirubin level that exceeds:

   A. 10 mg/dl term newborn

   B. 13 mg/dl term newborn

   C. 5 mg/dl term newborn

   D. 5 mg/dl term newborn

10. Which adaptation in the newborn is unrelated to cold stress?

    A. Hypoglycemia

    B. Increased oxygen consumption

    C. Increased metabolic acidosis

    D. Decreased lactic acid production

11. The primary heat production mechanism in the neonate is:

    A. Brown adipose tissue metabolism

    B. Shivering

    C. Sweating

    D. Decreasing oxygen consumption

12. Which of the following is unrelated to polycythemia?

    A. Cyanosis

    B. Transient tachypnea

    C. Jaundice

    D. Fever

Assessment of Risk in the Term Newborn

Knowledge regarding expected transition events, risk factors, newborn assessment and nursing care is therefore essential for neonatal nurses.

Susan Bakewell-Sachs
Valerie D. Shaw
Amy L. Tashman

Introduction

The newborn infant experiences many physiologic changes in the transition from fetal to extrauterine life. Changes in organ system functions and reorganization of metabolic processes require the establishment of pulmonary gas exchange, an adult cardiovascular pattern and a stable serum glucose level. The newborn must also maintain body temperature in this new environment and break down excess red blood cells. While the majority of term newborns achieve physiologic homeostasis without complications, assessment and monitoring of neonatal adaptation is essential for early identification of complications such as cold stress, hypoglycemia, infection, polycythemia and hyperbilirubinemia. Vitamin K, eye prophylaxis and routine screening for metabolic diseases are aspects of prevention and early identification of conditions that threaten the health and well-being of newborns. The perinatal history, including the maternal medical history and both antepartal and intrapartal data, gives the neonatal nurse important baseline information regarding potential risks for the newborn. Anthropometric, gestational age and physical assessment data, along with newborn behavior patterns, provide further evidence of risk and well-being. Nursing management during the early newborn period includes identification of risk factors, assessment, monitoring and intervention during hospitalization and postdischarge followup. Knowledge regarding expected transition events, risk factors, newborn assessment and nursing care is therefore essential for neonatal nurses.

Cardiovascular Adaptation

Successful transition to extrauterine life requires cardiopulmonary adaptation both from placental to pulmonary gas exchange and from fetal to adult circulation. Due to placental oxygenation and metabolic activities, the fetal lungs are essentially nonfunctional and the fetal liver is only partially functional. These organs consequently do not require large quantities of blood flow in utero. The placenta, however, must be highly perfused. Therefore, the route of fetal circulation differs from neonatal and adult circulation.

Oxygenated blood returns to the fetus from the placenta through the placental vein, mostly bypassing the liver via the ductus venosus (40% to 60%) and entering the inferior vena cava (IVC) (Blackburn & Loper, 1992). Most of the blood entering the right atrium from the IVC (50% to 60%) is then shunted across the right atrium through the foramen ovale directly into the left atrium. The aligned positioning of the IVC and the foramen ovale directs oxygenated blood from the placenta to the left side of the heart, bypassing the right side. Blood is then pumped by the left ventricle into the ascending aorta to supply the coronary, carotid and subclavian arteries.

Deoxygenated blood entering the right atrium from the superior vena cava (SVC) mixes somewhat with oxygenated blood from the IVC and is directed downward through the tricuspid valve into the right ventricle. From the right ventricle it is pumped into the pulmonary artery, where the majority (60%) is shunted across the ductus arteriosus into the descending aorta and through the umbilical arteries into the placenta. Deoxygenated blood is thereby shunted toward the placenta. Shunting of blood through the ductus venosus (liver to IVC), and the foramen ovale (right to the left atrium), directs blood with the highest oxygen content to the coronary arteries and brain, while the ductus arteriosus (pulmonary artery to descending aorta) directs the deoxygenated blood toward the placenta.

The shunting of blood flow in fetal circulation is accomplished by low resistance of the systemic and placental circulations and high resistance of the pulmonary vasculature. Pulmonary vascular resistance (PVR) greatly exceeds systemic resistance. As a result of the high PVR and the low systemic vascular resistance (SVR), only 5% to 10% of the cardiac output flows to the lungs (Blackburn & Loper, 1992).

Pulmonary Adaptation

Transition to extrauterine life requires aeration of the lungs with the conversion from placental to pulmonary gas exchange. This process occurs immediately at delivery. Clamping of the cord at birth removes the large, low-resistance placental circulation and decreases the neonate's intravascular space. There is a rapid rise in SVR

with the loss of the placenta, an initial drop in PVR as a result of expansion of the lungs and a significant rise in oxygen concentration (Blackburn & Loper, 1992). The increase in oxygen concentration causes vasodilatation of the pulmonary vascular bed and a significant increase in pulmonary blood flow. The rise in SVR increases the pressure in the left atrium, and the drop in PVR reduces the pressure in the right atrium, resulting in the combined effect of pressure closure of the foramen ovale. The ductus arteriosus begins to constrict almost immediately, in response to the rise in oxygen concentration; however, it may remain patent for several hours to days, permitting some left-to-right shunting (as opposed to right-to-left shunting during fetal life) from the aorta to the pulmonary artery. During the time the ductus arteriosus remains patent, a murmur may be heard on auscultation at the area of the second intercostal space, left sternal border. The murmur may be intermittent and then disappear entirely with no clinical signs associated with a persistently patent ductus arteriosus. Closure of the ductus arteriosus is also linked to a decreased level of circulating prostaglandin E2 (PGE2) following birth. Prostaglandins are metabolized in the lungs, a process that is greatly enhanced after birth as a result of increased pulmonary blood flow (Kirsten, 1996). Functional closure of the ductus arteriosus is usually accomplished within the first 24 to 96 hours after delivery; however, anatomic closure may take weeks or months (Kirsten, 1996).

The fetal lungs secrete fetal lung fluid (FLF) throughout gestation, at term yielding 10 to 25 ml/kg of body weight, which must be expelled or absorbed at birth (Blackburn & Loper, 1992). As gestation progresses closer to term, the lungs become less secretory. Early

Nurses should remain cognizant of limitations of the purpose and meaning of the Apgar score...

theories of FLF removal emphasized the thoracic squeeze during vaginal birth, especially as an explanation for retained FLF following cesarean birth (Nelson & Emery, 1993). Later studies emphasized the importance of labor, and concomitant catecholamine release, as important stimuli for the lungs to stop secreting lung fluid (Bland, 1992; Copper & Goldenberg, 1990). Neonates born via elective cesarean delivery have lower levels of catecholamines than neonates born vaginally or neonates subjected to a trial of labor but born by cesarean for reasons other than fetal distress (Falconer & Lake, 1982). This knowledge helps to explain why transient tachypnea of the newborn (TTN) is more commonly seen in infants born via elective cesarean who do not get the benefit of labor (Haywood, Coghill, Carlo, & Ross, 1993). Fetal lung fluid that remains after birth is removed via the circulatory and lymphatic systems as evidenced by distention of the interstitial spaces and lymphatics during the first five to six hours of life and

an increase in pulmonary lymph flow (Blackburn & Loper, 1992). During this time crackles may be auscultated across the newborn's lung fields.

Apgar Scoring

The Apgar score, an initial assessment of infant well-being, is used to assess the newborn's condition during the first minutes of transition to extrauterine life. The score evaluates five physiologic signs (heart rate, respiratory rate, color, tone and response to stimulation) at one and five minutes of life, assigning each a score of zero, one or two for a possible total score of zero to 10 (Apgar, 1953) (see Figure 1). Multiple factors can influence the Apgar score, including, but not limited to, gestational age, congenital malformations, maternal medications, infection, brainstem dysfunction and inconsistency among observers (American Academy of Pediatrics & American College of Obstetricians and Gynecologists, 1996; Carter, Haverkamp, & Merenstein, 1993; Nelson & Emery, 1993).

Figure 1. The Apgar Score			
	0	**1**	**2**
Heart Rate, beats/min.	Absent	Slow (< 100)	>100
Respirations	Absent	Weak cry, hypoventilation	Good, strong cry
Muscle Tone	Limp	Some flexion	Active motion
Reflex Irritability	No response	Grimace	Cry or active withdrawal
Color	Blue or pale	Body pink, extremities blue	Completely pink

Note. Adapted from "Use and Abuse of the Apgar Score" from the American Academy of Pediatrics, Committee on Fetus and Newborn, and American College of Obstetricians and Gynecologists, Committee on Obstetric Practice, *Pediatrics*, 1996, 98, 141-142. © 1996 by AAP and ACOG. Adapted with permission.

The Apgar score provides an assessment of the neonate's transition to extrauterine life; however, the decision to initiate resuscitation is not delayed until determination of the one-minute Apgar score (Bloom, Cropley, & AHA/AAP, 1995).

Evaluation of the need to initiate and/or continue resuscitation is based on assessment of respirations, heart rate, or color and, when indicated, interventions are immediately initiated. The Apgar score should be assigned at one and five minutes of age during a resuscitation and, when the score is less than seven, additional scores should be obtained every five minutes for up to 20 minutes (Bloom, Cropley, & AHA/AAP, 1995).

The Apgar score gained notoriety as a means to diagnose perinatal asphyxia and predict neonatal and long-term outcomes. Until 1993, the ICDM-9 codes included the use of Apgar scores with "severe birth asphyxia" coded for a five-minute Apgar score of four to seven (Carter, et al., 1993). This prevailed despite strong and consistent research evidence that one-minute Apgar scores of zero to three do not correlate with future outcomes, and scores of four to seven have no correlation with cerebral palsy (Carter, et al., 1993). Low Apgar scores are not diagnostic of hypoxia, acidosis or asphyxia. Low Apgar scores of zero to three that persist at 10, 15 and 20 minutes, however, have been shown to correlate with increased mortality and a greater likelihood of neurologic morbidity in infants who survive. Nurses should remain cognizant of limitations of the purpose and meaning of the Apgar score and educate families who may misunderstand its purpose. Nurses involved in performing Apgar assessments must be objective and appropriately and accurately assign scores (Letko, 1996).

Perinatal Asphyxia

Perinatal asphyxia is of concern to perinatal health professionals and to families; additionally, it has been a diagnosis for litigation in cases of cerebral palsy and mental retardation. Defining asphyxia, preventing it, and correlating it with specific and sensitive clinical measures have been the focus of clinical and research efforts.

The biochemical hallmarks of perinatal asphyxia include profound metabolic or mixed acidosis, hypoxemia and hypercarbia. Fetal asphyxia primarily occurs as a result of impaired uteroplacental exchange, related to such conditions as impaired uterine blood flow, maternal hypoxia, maternal hypotension, placental insufficiency or abruption, and compression of the umbilical cord (Williams, Mallard, Tan, & Gluckman, 1993). Neonatal asphyxia can present in relation to a variety of causes as well, including birth trauma, failed initiation of respiration, respiratory distress syndrome and apnea. The healthy term fetus or newborn is able to reduce overall oxygen consumption and protect vital organs such as the brain and the heart in response to hypoxemia and the threat of asphyxia. Tissue damage results when the severity of inadequate perfusion overwhelms the compensatory mechanisms. Such damage is more accurately termed hypoxic-ischemic, since hypoxia and ischemia constitute the underlying mechanisms for injury. If adequate oxygenation and perfusion are quickly restored, injury is reversible; if the event is too severe or prolonged, tissue damage will occur (Williams, et al., 1993).

Acute clinical sequelae involving multiple organ systems in the newborn period have been described in relation to perinatal asphyxia. Neurologic signs in the term infant may include seizures;

The healthy term fetus or newborn is able to reduce overall oxygen consumption and protect vital organs ... in response to hypoxemia...

abnormal respiratory patterns with apnea and respiratory arrest; an apparent state of hyperalertness; jitteriness, posturing and movement disorders, impaired suck, swallow, gag and feeding; abnormal eye movements and pupillary responses; hypotonia and lethargy; and a bulging anterior fontanel (Carter, et al., 1993; Witt, 1991). Neonatal seizures may also occur secondary to intracranial hemorrhage, hypoglycemia, hypocalcemia, neurodevelopmental abnormalities and drug withdrawal (Volpe, 1987). Pulmonary effects may include pulmonary hypertension, surfactant deficiency and meconium aspiration syndrome. Renal effects include oliguria, hematuria, proteinuria, renal failure and renal vein thrombosis.

Described acute cardiovascular effects include tricuspid insufficiency, myocardial necrosis, and cardiogenic

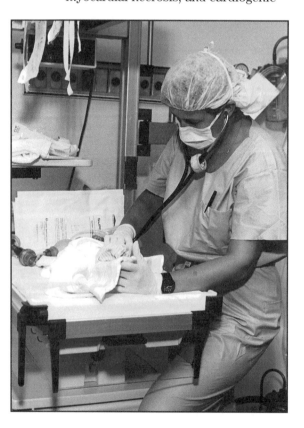

shock/hypotension. Necrotizing enterocolitis and hepatic dysfunction are gastrointestinal effects, and hematologic sequelae include thrombocytopenia and disseminated intravascular coagulopathy. Perinatal asphyxia with severe hypoxic-ischemic encephalopathy (HIE) can result in death. Intensive care and intervention offers the necessary support during the period of acute multisystem dysfunction and failure. If the infant survives the acute phase, long-term followup is necessary to monitor central nervous system function for residual sequelae (Carter, et al., 1993).

The term "perinatal asphyxia" has been used inconsistently and, based on long-term outcomes, inaccurately as a diagnosis. The Committees on Maternal-Fetal Medicine and Fetus and Newborn of the American College of Obstetricians and Gynecologists (ACOG), and the American Academy of Pediatrics (AAP) have, therefore, defined four essential criteria that must all be present when perinatal asphyxia that has the potential for neurologic sequelae occurs (1992, 1996). These include:

1. Profound metabolic or mixed acidemia (pH < 7.00) on an umbilical artery sample

2. Persistent low Apgar score of zero to three for greater than five minutes

3. Clinical neurologic sequelae in the immediate neonatal period, such as seizures, hypotonia, coma

4. Clinical evidence of multiorgan system dysfunction in the immediate neonatal period.

All of these criteria must be present to conclude that perinatal asphyxia has occurred.

Management at Delivery

Delivery room management is a vital aspect of perinatal services, including appropriate personnel, equipment, education and planning. Since six percent of all newborns can be expected to require some form of resuscitation, all health care personnel who attend deliveries should be prepared to provide appropriate intervention (Leuthner, Jansen, & Hageman, 1994).

The American Heart Association (AHA) and the American Academy of Pediatrics (AAP) cosponsor the Neonatal Resuscitation Program (NRP), a program that evolved from initial guidelines developed by the Emergency Cardiac Care Committee of the AHA in 1979. The goal of the national education program is to educate health care practitioners so that every delivery area is stocked with the necessary equipment, and every delivery can be attended by at least one person skilled in resuscitating infants at birth (Bloom, Cropley, AHA/AAP, 1995; Leuthner, et al., 1994). All NRP course materials can be ordered from the American Academy of Pediatrics, Publications Department, P.O. Box 927, Elk Grove Village, IL 60009-0927, 800-433-9016.

Effects of Anesthesia/Analgesia on the Neonate

Nearly all of the medications used for anesthesia and analgesia during labor for pain control cross the placenta and enter the fetal circulation. Effects on the fetus and newborn must be considered when deciding which drugs to use in labor (Hughes & DeVore, 1993). The impact of drugs used in labor must also be considered when assessing the neonate's transition to extrauterine life.

Analgesia refers to relief of pain without loss of consciousness. Classifications of analgesic drugs usually used during labor and delivery include narcotic agonist and mixed narcotic agonist/ antagonist compounds (Felblinger & Weitkamp, 1993). Narcotic agonists, widely used to provide pain relief during labor and delivery, readily cross the placental blood barrier, causing central nervous system (CNS) depression in the newborn. The neonate born within one to two hours of a narcotic dosage to the mother will initially appear sleepy with poor respiratory effort and may require resuscitative measures at delivery. Naloxone (Narcan), a narcotic antagonist, may be administered to the newborn to reduce respiratory depression. Narcan is contraindicated when the mother is a narcotic addict, however, as it may precipitate acute withdrawal in the neonate (Goldsmith & Starrett, 1991). Narcotic agonist/antagonist compounds provide pain relief and counteract narcotic-associated respiratory depression.

Sedatives and tranquilizers are also used during labor (Felblinger & Weitkamp, 1993). Sedatives do not relieve pain, but can be used in early labor to reduce anxiety and facilitate rest and sleep. Tranquilizers are used to increase maternal relaxation and are given with narcotics to potentiate narcotic effectiveness. Sedatives and tranquilizers can cause maternal hypotension and reduce uteroplacental circulation. Newborns may demonstrate hypotonia, drowsiness and diminished feeding. Table 1 presents commonly used analgesics, mixed combination drugs, and sedatives with possible neonatal effects.

The impact of drugs used in labor must also be considered when assessing the neonate's transition to extrauterine life.

Table 1. Drugs Used for Analgesia and Anesthesia During Labor and Delivery

Drug	Possible Adverse Effects in Newborn
Narcotic Agonists Meperidine (Demerol) Oxymorphine (Numorphan)	CNS depression with respiratory depression if maternal administration 1 to 2 hours before birth; mild behavioral depression
Narcotic Agonist/Antagonist Combinations Butorphanol tartrate (Stadol)	CNS depression; mild behavioral depression; similar to meperidine
Nalbuphine (Nubain)	Respiratory depression, apnea, bradycardia, cardia arrhythmias
Tranquilizers (Sedative-Hypnotics) Promethazine (Phenergan) Hydroxyzine (Vistaril)	Possible hypotonia, hypothermia, reduced feeding, drowsiness
Regional Anesthetic Agents Chlorprocaine (Nesacaine) Lidocaine (Xylocaine) Mepivacaine (Carbocaine) Bupivacaine (Marcaine)	CNS depression, neurobehavioral changes, jaundice, hypotonia
General Anesthetic Agents Halothane, Enflurane, Thiopental Sodium	CNS depression, short-term behavioral changes

Note. Adapted from K.C. Hanold, V.H. Kemp, and T.P. Nelms. In C.A. Kenner & A. MacLaren (Eds.), *Essentials of Maternal and Neonatal Nursing*, 1996, 220. © 1996 by Springhouse. Adapted with permission

Anesthesia produces loss of sensation and, with general anesthesia, loss of consciousness. Regional anesthetic agents, or blocks, provide pain relief by blocking the nerve impulses to a particular area. Epidural and spinal blocks are common regional anesthetics used in labor and delivery. The main adverse effect of regional anesthesia is maternal hypotension with the potential to cause fetal distress. General anesthesia is usually only used for emergency cesarean delivery or other surgical intervention and can cause fetal CNS depression and neonatal behavioral changes.

Neurobehavioral effects of anesthetics on the neonate are documented. When assessed on scales such as the Neonatal Behavioral Assessment Scale (NBAS) or the Early Neonatal Neurobehavioral Scale (ENNS), infants of mothers who received either narcotic analgesia or epidural anesthesia have been shown to perform less well on tests of muscle tone, alertness and motor skills than those whose mothers did not receive any anesthesia or analgesia; however, these effects are transient and resolve themselves within the first few days of life (Goldsmith & Starrett, 1991).

Respiratory Distress

Respiratory distress is one of the most common neonatal complications. It results in a decreased ability to ensure oxygenation and carbon dioxide exchange, affecting all body organs and tissues if prolonged (Nash, 1996). Respiratory distress occurs in the presence of obstruction or malformation, develops as a complication to transition to extrauterine life, or occurs in the presence of other medical or systemic problems.

Risk Factors. Since a number of perinatal conditions and events enhance the risk for respiratory distress in the newborn, a complete perinatal history is imperative (see Table 2).

The three most common respiratory conditions that result in respiratory distress in the term newborn are pneumonia, Transient Tachypnea of the Newborn (TTN) and Meconium Aspiration Syndrome (MAS). Table 3 presents an overview of these respiratory problems.

Respiratory distress is one of the most common neonatal complications.

Table 2. Clinical Correlates of Perinatal History	
History	**Associated Respiratory Disease**
Premature Birth Maternal diabetes Maternal hemorrhage Perinatal asphyxia	RDS
Multiple gestation	RDS more common in second twin
Postmature Birth Nonreassuring fetal heart rate Meconium-stained amniotic fluid Perinatal asphyxia	Meconium Aspiration Syndrome (MAS) Persistent pulmonary pattern hypertension
Oligohydramnios	Pulmonary hypoplasia
Polyhydramnios Choking on feeding Drooling	Tracheoesophageal fistula with esophageal atresia
Cesarean birth	Transient Tachypnea of the Newborn (TTN)
Prolonged rupture of membranes Maternal fever	Pneumonia/sepsis
Traumatic delivery	Poor respiratory effort
Narcotics in labor	Poor respiratory effort

Note. Adapted from C. Kenner, A. Brueggemeyer, and L. P. Gunderson, *Comprehensive Neonatal Nursing*, 1993. © 1993 by W. B. Saunders. Adapted by permission.

Table 3. Respiratory Problems in the Neonate			
	TTN	**Aspiration Syndrome**	**Strep and Pneumococcal Pneumonitis Sepsis**
Gestational Age	Near-Term and Term	Term, Post-Term, SGA, Near-Term	Near-Term and Term
Etiology	Delayed resorption of fetal lung fluid	Aspiration of amniotic fluid and debris Purulent fluid Blood Meconium	B-Hemolytic Strep Groups B & D Pneumococcus
Contributing Factors	C-section Neonatal depression secondary to maternal drugs	Intrauterine/Perinatal stress Any predisposing factor associated with fetal distress, i.e., postmaturity placental dysfunction complicated delivery	Maternal colonization
Complications	Just about none	Pneumothorax Pneumomediastinum Persistent fetal circulation Hypoxic & Ischemic damage to other organs (CNS, kidneys, liver, etc.)	DIC Shock Hypoperfusion
Clinical	Tachypnea usually without dyspnea Minimal cyanosis Good gas exchange Early onset	Often postmature Tachypnea Often requires high O_2 concentration to relieve cyanosis Retractions Rales Grunting Flaring Wheezing	Latent period then acute picture Respiratory distress Apnea Shock Poor capillary refill Neutropenia or leukocytosis in over 2/3
X-ray	Overaeration Fluid in fissures of lung Interstitial edema Cardiomegaly	Overaeration Diffuse fluffy (alveolar) or streaky (interstitial) densities	Underaeration
Clinical	Resolved in 24 to 48 hrs No residual	Usually resolved by one week Increased PVR may result from hypoxia and acidosis leading to PFC Often have CNS damage Death may result from an inability to oxygenate	Early onset: pneumonia sepsis shock; DIC death in 25%-50%

Note. Compiled from "Complications of Respiratory Management" by S. M. Southwell. In C. Kenner, A. Brueggemeyer, and L.P. Gunderson, *Comprehensive Neonatal Nursing*, 1993, Philadelphia: W.B. Saunders Company 1993. Reprinted by permission.

Clinical Signs and Symptoms. The term newborn with upper airway congestion and minor airway infections may experience tremendous pulmonary resistance, placing the newborn at risk for increased work of breathing, muscle fatigue and respiratory failure (Blackburn & Loper, 1992). Trauma or infection of the upper airway passages may result in edema, with subsequent obstruction and decreased airflow. Constriction in the airways of a term newborn results in nasal flaring, retractions and tachypnea (Blackburn & Loper, 1992). Chest wall retractions (subcostal, intercostal, suprasternal) and use of accessory muscles are evident when there is increased work of breathing, indicating a primary pulmonary disorder (Blackburn & Loper, 1992). Unequal breath sounds, diminished air entry and adventitious sounds such as crackles, wheezes and rhonchi provide further evidence of a pulmonary problem.

Care of a newborn with respiratory distress requires basic understanding of the causative factors of the disease processes. Each of the most common conditions will be reviewed.

Pneumonia

Pneumonias may be of viral, bacterial or other infectious origin. Transmission can occur transplacentally or by ascending infection following rupture of the membranes (see Perinatal Infections). Pneumonia-producing organisms most commonly associated with maternal amnionitis include Group B Streptococcus, Escherichia Coli and Haemophilus influenzae (Haywood, et al., 1993). Less commonly, Streptococcus viridans and Listeria are involved. The resultant inflammatory process associated with pneumonia disrupts the normal barrier function of the pulmonary endothelium, leading to abnormal protein permeability and edema of lung tissue (Nash, 1996). Tachypnea, prolonged grunting and retractions beyond the immediate transition period, as well as temperature instability in the term newborn, warrant further evaluation.

Transient Tachypnea of the Newborn

Transient tachypnea of the newborn occurs in approximately 11 per 1,000 live births (Whitsett, Pryhuber, Rice, Werner, & Wert, 1994). Contributing factors include maternal oversedation and cesarean birth (without a trial of labor). Delayed absorption of fetal lung fluid is considered to be the underlying etiology.

Initially, the newborn is asymptomatic; however, symptoms such as expiratory grunting, flaring of the nares and mild cyanosis are exhibited shortly after birth. Tachypnea usually occurs by six hours of age, with a respiratory rate as high as 140 breaths per minute. The newborn with TTN usually recovers within 24 to 48 hours with no major sequelae. Management consists of ruling out other causes of RDS and maintaining adequate oxygenation.

Meconium Aspiration Syndrome

Meconium stained amniotic fluid may be present when the fetus has experienced hypoxia in utero. Meconium in the amniotic fluid occurs in approximately 10% of all deliveries. Risk factors include: postmaturity, small for gestational age, fetal distress due to maternal hypertension, anemia or chronic disease. Approximately 4% of newborns with meconium stained amniotic fluid will develop Meconium Aspiration Syndrome (Whitsett, et al., 1994).

Meconium Aspiration Syndrome is the most common respiratory distress syndrome in the neonate. Meconium that is aspirated below the vocal cords and into the trachea causes partial or com-

Care of a newborn with respiratory distress requires basic understanding of the causative factors of the disease processes.

27

Neonatal hypo-glycemia can be asymptomatic, symptomatic or life-threatening...

plete obstruction of the terminal airways and air sacs. Meconium creates a ball-valve effect, in which air enters the lower airways on inspiration but is trapped on exhalation. This results in overdistension of the airways leading to alveolar rupture and air leaks. In addition, aspiration of products that are foreign substrate in the lungs leads to an inflammatory process (pneumonitis) in the terminal airways and air sacs. These changes in the airway result in increased pulmonary vascular resistance and can lead to persistent pulmonary hypertension of the newborn (PPHN) (Eichenwald, 1991; Usta, Mercer, & Sibai, 1995).

Neonatal Hypoglycemia

The interruption of the transport of nutrients from mother to baby following cord clamping forces the newborn to mobilize fuels to meet the metabolic demands of vital organs. The newborn must adjust to this cessation of the maternal glucose supply, while responding to an increased demand for energy secondary to changes in body temperature, the stress of labor and initiation of breathing (Girard & Narkewicz, 1992; Padbury & Ogata, 1992). Glucose, the primary fuel, is stored as glycogen in the liver (Girard & Narkewicz, 1992). During fetal life, glucose is diverted into glycogen storage in preparation for the immediate newborn period. Neonatal hypoglycemia occurs when expected metabolic adaptation is unable to maintain glucose homeostasis.

Neonatal hypoglycemia can be asymptomatic, symptomatic or life-threatening and has the potential for adverse neurologic sequelae such as seizures and learning disabilities (Cole, 1991). The risk of brain damage or developmental consequences may be related to the duration and severity of the hypoglycemia (Kleigman, 1993). Therefore, early assessment of new-

borns and early initiation of preventive measures are important.

There is no consensus regarding expected newborn blood glucose levels or the definition of hypoglycemia. Kalhan (1993) states that a full-term, healthy neonate maintains plasma glucose levels between 40 and 80 mg/dl during the first six hours of life, and that after 24 hours of life, normal plasma glucose levels range between 45 and 90 mg/dl. Hypoglycemia is difficult to define, in part, because there is no correlation between blood glucose levels and central nervous system effects (Cowett, 1992). A wide range of blood levels is used to define hypoglycemia by various authors and institutions. Clinically, a blood glucose of less than 40 mg/dl is commonly used to define hypoglycemia and initiate further evaluation and intervention (Cole, 1991). It is recommended that each institution establish guidelines for hypoglycemia screening in newborns (AAP/ACOG, 1992).

Glucose Physiology and Etiology of Hypoglycemia. Glucose homeostasis in the newborn depends on the initiation of several hormonal and metabolic changes. Catecholamine levels (primarily norepinephrine) increase after birth, in response to a drop in body temperature, causing an increase in glucagon levels. The elevated glucagon and norepinephrine levels initiate activation of glycogenolysis, the conversion of hepatic glycogen stores to glucose. The norepinephrine also initiates lipolysis, providing substrate for gluconeogenesis, the manufacture of glucose from noncarbohydrate sources such as protein and fat (Cornblath & Schwartz, 1993). The hormones that are involved in glucose balance can be classified as either lowering blood glucose or elevating blood glucose. Insulin is the glucose lowering hormone. Glucagon, epinephrine, gluco-corticoids and growth factor hormones are known as blood glucose elevating hormones. Glucagon promotes the conversion of glycogen to glucose when there is an immediate need for energy (Blackburn & Loper, 1992; Girard & Narkewicz, 1992). Hypoglycemia results from inadequate substrate supply, abnormal endocrine regulation of glucose metabolism and increased rate of glucose utilization (McGowan, Hagedorn, & Hay, 1993). Hyperinsulinemia and resultant hypo-glycemia in infants of diabetic mothers are believed to be related to poor maternal glucose control. According to Mehta, Woolton, Cheng, Penfold, Halliday, and Stacey (1987), infants of diabetic mothers (IDM) have a lower incidence of neonatal hypo-glycemia when their mothers are managed according to current practice guidelines. Other conditions that have been known to be associated with hypoglycemia due to hyperinsulinemia are syndromes such as Beckwith-Weidemann and islet cell dysregula-tion. Tocolytics used in the treatment of preterm labor can cause maternal hyperglycemia, leading to fetal hyper-insulinism and neonatal hypoglycemia (Karp, Scardino, & Butler, 1995).

Hypoglycemia has also been reported in infants born to preeclamptic moth-ers, in infants with hypothermia and infants with perinatal acidosis.

Newborn hypoglycemia may be cate-gorized as either transient or persis-tent. Transient hypoglycemia, the most common type of hypoglycemia in the newborn period, usually occurs within the first 48 hours of life but may not present until 72 hours of life or later in some infants (Kleigman, 1993; Pildes & Lilian, 1992). Persistent hypoglycemia is defined as hypoglycemia that does not resolve over several hours and may persist for days even with treat-ment. It can result from inborn errors of metabolism, hyperinsulinism sec-ondary to beta cell hyperplasia and endocrine disorders (McGowan, et al., 1993). Neonates developing hypo-glycemia in the first 24 hours of life typically have either a maternal history (e.g., infant of diabetic mother), physi-cal findings (e.g., intrauterine growth retardation, SGA, LGA), or evidence of stress (asphyxia, sepsis, hypothermia, respiratory distress), categorizing them as high-risk (Baird & Witt, 1996). Table 4 identifies etiologies and time course of neonatal hypoglycemia.

Table 4. Neonatal Hypoglycemia: Etiologies and Time Course		
Mechanism	**Clinical Setting**	**Expected Duration**
Decreased substrate availability	Intrauterine growth retardation	Transient
	Glycogen storage disease	Transient
	Inborn errors (e.g., fructose intolerance)	Persistent
Endocrine disturbances		
Hyperinsulinemia	Infant of a diabetic mother	Transient
	Beckwith-Wiedemann syndrome	Persistent
	Exchange transfusion	Transient
	Islet cell hyperplasia	Persistent
	Maternal tocolytic therapy	Transient
	Insulin-producing tumors	Persistent
	Excessive maternal fluid therapy in labor	Transient
Other endocrine disorders	Hypopituitarism	Persistent
	Hypothyroidism	Persistent
	Adrenal insufficiency	Persistent
Increased utilization	Perinatal asphyxia	Transient
	Hypothermia	Transient
Miscellaneous/ multiple mechanisms	Sepsis	Transient
	Congenital heart disease	Transient
	Polycythemia	Transient

Note. Adapted from "Glucose Homeostasis" by J. McGowan, M. Hagedorn, and W. Hay. In G. B. Merenstein and S. L. Gardner (Eds.), *Handbook of Neonatal Intensive Care* (3rd ed.), 1993, 229. © 1993 by Mosby. Adapted by permission.

Signs and Symptoms. In the newborn period, signs of hypoglycemia may be absent or subtle despite extremely low blood glucose levels. When the plasma glucose level reaches a concentration of approximately 40 mg/dl, signs and symptoms generally become apparent (Karp, et al., 1995). Signs and symptoms of neonatal hypoglycemia may include lethargy, apnea, cyanosis, hypothermia and seizures (Cole, 1991; Stokowski, 1992). Additional manifestations include sweating, tachycardia, jitteriness, muscle twitching, high-pitched cry, irregular respirations, difficulty in feeding and hunger (Cowett, 1992). If hypoglycemia remains untreated, manifestations of cerebral dysfunction such as irritability, seizures and coma develop, with resultant permanent central nervous system damage (see Table 5).

Table 5. Signs and Symptoms of Hypoglycemia		
Apnea	Hypothermia	Poor feeding
Abnormal cry	Hypotonia	Respiratory distress
Cardiac arrest	Irritability	Seizures
Cardiac failure	Jitters	Tachypnea
Cyanosis	Lethargy	Tremors

Note. Adapted from "Neonatal Glucose Screening" by P.B. Baird, and C.L. Witt, 1995, and Baird, et al., (1996). *Neonatal Network*, 15(7), 63-66. Used by permission.

Breast milk appears to be more ketogenic than formula and therefore breastfeeding is encouraged (Hawdon, Platt-Ward & Aynsley-Green, 1992).

Management of Neonatal Hypoglycemia. Anticipation and prevention are the goals of nursing management for hypoglycemia (Karp, et al., 1995). Infants at risk should be routinely assessed for clinical signs and have routine blood glucose screening. All newborns should be fed within the first two hours of life (breast or bottle) and early feedings should be considered for at-risk newborns (Nash, 1996). Maintaining an adequate thermal environment is critical in preventing an increase in metabolic demand due to hypothermia. A confirmed lab value indicative of hypoglycemia may be treated with a bolus of 2 ml/kg of $D_{10}W$ followed immediately by an infusion of 6 to 8mg/kg/min to maintain a blood glucose level above 40 mg/dl (Cowett, 1992; Downey & Cloherty, 1991; Karp, et al., 1995). Frequent monitoring of glucose level (chemstrip, lab analysis) and close observation of the state of hydration are critical (Downey & Cloherty, 1991). Once an adequate blood glucose level is achieved and maintained, it is not necessary to measure blood glucose concentration repeatedly unless there is a reduction in exogenous glucose supply (Hawdon & Ward, 1993). Significant changes in clinical condition or reduction in fluid or nutrient intake should be followed by blood glucose monitoring.

The introduction of enteral feedings, either breast milk or formula, is important in the management of neonatal hypoglycemia. Milk (breast or formula) provides more energy per ml than 10% dextrose and also supplies important non-glucose fuels, which are necessary in the glucose sparing role for neurologic function (Hawdon & Ward, 1993). Breast milk appears to be more ketogenic than formula and therefore breastfeeding is encouraged (Hawdon, Platt-Ward, & Aynsley-Green, 1992). Enteral feedings should not be discontinued or reduced when intravenous fluids are given. By maximizing enteral feeding intake and gradually reducing intravenous infusion rates, most newborns will achieve glucose homeostasis. Ongoing nursing assessment for signs and symptoms of hypoglycemia are imperative. In addition, respiratory distress can result in increased utilization of glucose with resultant lactic acidosis; therefore, the nurse should also assess the newborn for grunting, nasal flaring and intercostal retractions.

Parental involvement in the care of the newborn with hypoglycemia should be encouraged. The mother who wishes to breastfeed should be supported and encouraged to do so. For additional information on breastfeeding teaching, refer to the March of Dimes modules entitled *Breastfeeding the Healthy Newborn* and *Breastfeeding the Infant with Special Needs.*

Glucose Monitoring. Identification of infants with abnormal glucose states requires blood glucose screening. Several methods are employed to determine glucose levels in the neonate, all with advantages and disadvantages. Glucose reagent strips are commonly used for routine bedside screening. Results with this method are dependent on the hematocrit, have great variance and lack reproducibility, especially at levels less than 50 mg/dl (Cornblath, Schwartz, Aynsley-Green, & Lloyd, 1990). Accuracy is dependent upon use of proper technique, following the manufacturer's instructions. A drop of blood is placed to cover the test pad; after a designated time, the strip is rinsed and the resultant color is visually compared to a color chart, signifying a glucose range (Karp, et al., 1995). For longevity and accuracy, the reagent strips must be stored in airtight containers and shelf-life dates must be adhered to. Isopropyl alcohol left on the skin prior to puncture to obtain blood can cause a false elevation in the results (Cornblath, et al., 1990). Reflectance meters and glucometers eliminate some human variables

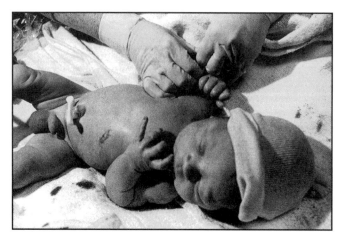

(comparing colors, appropriate timing, wiping techniques), which may make these instruments somewhat more reliable than reagent strips (Baird & Witt, 1996). A glucometer requires that a drop of blood be placed on a reagent strip or test spot. Most meters use an electronic "red eye" to measure the amount of glucose in the blood. When using a glucometer, the blood-saturated reagent strip is placed into a meter, which measures the amount of light reflected from the sample and converts this to a glucose value (Karp, et al., 1995). Manufacturer's instructions must be followed carefully to avoid inaccurate readings and glucometers must be routinely calibrated to ensure accuracy. Glucose reflectance meters may be unreliable in evaluation of capillary blood glucose concentration; for example, when the neonate's hematocrit is over 55%, readings tend to be low, while hematocrits below 35% tend to result in falsely high readings (Lin, et al., 1989). The One Touch II hospital system, set in the neonatal mode, accurately determines the blood glucose levels of neonatal capillary whole blood (Altimier & Roberts, 1996). The benefit of utilizing the One Touch II meter is that it gives immediate quantitative results not subject to observer bias as seen with other methods. However, the most accurate means of measuring blood glucose is through laboratory analysis of serum (Cornblath & Schwartz, 1993). Whatever method is used in the nursery, abnormal results must be confirmed by laboratory serum analysis.

Neonatal Hyperglycemia

Hyperglycemia in the newborn is usually defined as a blood glucose level over 125 mg/dl. Hyperglycemia most often occurs in preterm newborns; however, it may occur in term neonates with sepsis, decreased insulin sensitivity or infants with respiratory distress (Amspacher, 1992; Stiles & Cloherty, 1991). It is typically asymptomatic, detected on routine laboratory screening. Hyperglycemia may result in osmotic diuresis, in which fluids are drawn from the intracellular to the extracellular space resulting in dehydration (Amspacher, 1992; Gomella, 1992). Such fluid shifts may be a risk factor for intracranial bleeding. As a followup to management of hyperglycemia, monitoring of the blood glucose level and urine assessment for osmotic diuresis are necessary.

Thermoregulation in the Newborn

Thermoregulation and prevention of cold stress are critical elements of nursing care at the time of birth. Thermoregulation is the balance between heat production and heat loss, with the goal of maintaining thermal equilibrium. The fetus moves from a warm, wet intrauterine environment to a cool, dry extrauterine environment. The newborn experiences rapid heat loss after birth, primarily through evaporation, with a fall in temperature of 2° C to 3° C (Blackburn & Loper, 1992). Cold stress occurs when heat loss overwhelms the newborn's ability to produce heat. Poor thermal stability in the neonate is primarily due to excessive heat loss rather than impaired heat production. During the first four hours after birth, the newborn is at greatest risk of becoming cold stressed (Bliss-Holtz, 1993). Nursing interventions to minimize heat loss at birth include: thoroughly drying the newborn; wrapping the infant in a

warm, dry blanket; covering the dried newborn's head with an insulated cap; and facilitating skin-to-skin contact with the mother. Placing the infant on a prewarmed radiant warmer or in a prewarmed incubator, and using prewarmed equipment will further reduce heat losses. The expected rectal temperature for a newborn is 36.5° C to 37°C (97.6° F to 98.6° F) and skin temperature is 36.0° C to 36.5° C (97.1° F to 97.8° F) (Blackburn & Loper, 1992). Table 6 provides an overview of sources of heat loss, overheating and nursing interventions.

Head Covering. Head coverings of different materials are frequently used to minimize heat loss in newborns. Rationale for this practice lies in the knowledge that the newborn's head comprises 21 percent of the total body surface area. In addition, 44% of heat production in the newborn takes place in the brain (D'Apolito, 1994). Stockinette or cotton tubular material, commonly used in hospitals to make caps for newborns, has generally been found to be ineffective in reducing heat loss (Coles & Valman, 1979; Greer, 1988; Stothers, 1981), even when doubled. More effective head coverings include: 1) wool with a gauze and cotton lining; 2) Thinsulate (polyolefin microfibers commonly used to manufacture winter outerwear); and 3) cotton/polyester fill, and terry cloth (Coles & Valman, 1979; Greer, 1988; Rowe, Weinberg, & Andrews, 1983; Stothers, 1981). Thinsulate hats can reduce heat loss by 65% in full-term newborns (Rowe, et al., 1983).

Thermoregulation and prevention of cold stress are critical elements of nursing care at the time of birth.

Table 6. Sources of Heat Loss, Overheating and Nursing Interventions

Mechanisms	Sources of Heat Loss/Overheating	Interventions
Evaporation	Wet body surface and hair at delivery and with bathing	Thoroughly dry infant, especially the head, immediately after birth with a warm blanket Use insulated caps or hooded blankets Replace wet blankets with warm, dry ones Place dried infant skin-to-skin on mother's chest and cover with warmed blanket Maintain warm environment Delay initial bath until body temperature has stabilized Bathe in warm, draft-free environment and dry immediately; bathe under a radiant warmer
Conduction	Cool mattress, blanket, scale, table, equipment or clothing	Place warm blankets on scales, X-ray plates, other surfaces in direct contact with infant Preheat blankets, clothing, radiant warmer and equipment before use Heating pads, hot water bottles, chemical bags Transport infants in prewarmed incubators Avoid placing infant on any surface that is warmer than the infant
Convection	Cool air temperature in room, hallways or outside air	Maintain room temperature at levels adequate to provide a safe thermal environment for infant (72° to 76° F) Swaddle with warm blankets (except when under radiant warmer), use insulated caps or hooded blankets
	Convective air-flow incubator	Monitor incubator air temperature to avoid temperatures warmer than the infant's body temperature
	Drafts from air vents, windows, doors, heaters, fans, air conditioners	Place infants away from air vents, drafts and other sources of moving air currents Use side guards on radiant warmers to decrease cross current air flow across infant
	Cold oxygen flow (especially near facial thermal receptors)	Use warm and humidified oxygen; minimize use of cool, dry free-flow oxygen
	Placement near cold or hot external windows or walls, placement in direct sunlight	Place incubators, cribs and radiant warmers away from external walls and windows, direct sunlight Use thermal shades on external windows
Radiation	Cold incubator walls	Prewarm incubators, radiant warmers, heat shields
	Heat lamps	Avoid use whenever possible; if used, monitor temperature every 10-15 minutes to avoid burns

Note. Adapted from "Thermoregulation" by S.T. Blackburn and D.L. Loper. In S.T. Blackburn and D.L. Loper, (Eds.), *Maternal, Fetal, and Neonatal Physiology: A Clinical Perspective*, 1992, 691. © 1992 by W.B. Saunders. Reprinted by permission.

Mechanisms of Heat Transfer. Heat transfer occurs between warmer and cooler areas when a difference or gradient exists. The two routes of heat transfer relating to body heat exchange are the internal and external gradients (Blackburn & Loper, 1992). The internal gradient refers to heat transfer between the warmer body core and the cooler body surface, determined physiologically by regulation of blood flow. Peripheral vasoconstriction reduces blood flow to the skin surface to minimize heat loss and vasodilation increases blood flow to the skin to maximize dissipation of excess heat. Factors that influence heat transfer across the internal gradient include the amount of insulating subcutaneous fat and the surface-to-body-mass ratio. The newborn has a thinner layer of subcutaneous fat and a thin epidermis, with blood vessels closer to the skin than those of an adult. In addition, the newborn infant has a larger surface-to-body ratio. The infant's body weight is 5% of the adult's and its body surface area is 15% of the adult's, placing the full-term infant at risk for three to four times more heat loss than an adult (Bullock, 1992).

The external gradient refers to heat transfer between the surface of the body and the environment. The four mechanisms of heat loss from the surface of the body are radiation, conduction, convection and evaporation. Factors that influence heat transfer across the external gradient in newborns include exposed skin surface area, subcutaneous tissue thickness, the difference or gradient in temperature between the body surface and the surrounding air and surfaces near the newborn, and air currents (Blackburn & Loper, 1992; TePas, 1988).

Neonatal Heat Production. Three mechanisms of human heat production are voluntary muscle activity, involuntary muscle activity (shivering), and nonshivering thermogenesis. Shivering is the main source of heat production in adults and nonshivering thermogenesis is the major response to cold in the newborn (Whatley & Schlosser, 1992). Newborns achieve some heat production through increased muscle activity in the form of restlessness, crying and agitation. Heat conservation is attempted through assuming a flexed posture to decrease surface area and through peripheral vasoconstriction (Le Blanc, 1992). The neonate accomplishes nonshivering or chemical thermogenesis primarily through brown adipose tissue (BAT) metabolism. Brown fat, deposited after 28 weeks gestation and up to five weeks after birth, is a highly vascular form of adipose tissue surrounding the scapulae, kidneys, adrenal glands, head, neck, heart, great vessels and axillary regions (Auvenshine & Enriquez, 1990; Blackburn & Loper, 1992) (see Figure 2). Brown fat accounts for 2% to 7% of the infant's weight (Bruck, 1978). In response to a decrease in skin temperature, thermal receptors transmit impulses to the posterior hypothalamus. The sympathetic nervous system is stimulated, resulting in norepinephrine release in the BAT (Blackburn & Loper, 1992). Norepinephrine activates lipase, which in turn leads to lipolysis and fatty acid oxidation, resulting in heat production. The heat is transferred to the blood perfusing the brown fat and nearby tissues. Physiologic consequences of BAT metabolism are presented in Figure 3. The cold-stressed newborn may deplete glycogen stores and develop hypoglycemia, develop metabolic acidosis secondary to anaerobic metabolism and fatty acid release, and show signs of respiratory distress.

Figure 2. Brown Adipose Tissue

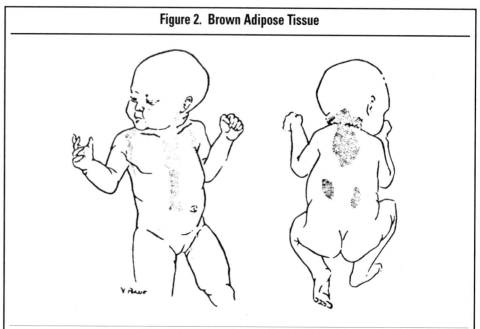

Note. From "The Structure and Function of Brown Adipose Tissue in the Neonate" by V. Davis, *JOGNN*, 1980, 9(6), 369. Illustrations by V. Poazio. Used by permission.

Figure 3. Sequelae of BAT Metabolism

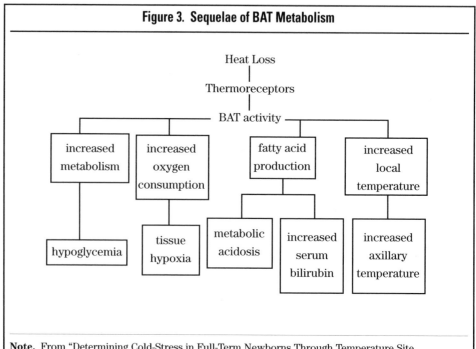

Note. From "Determining Cold-Stress in Full-Term Newborns Through Temperature Site Comparisons" by J. Bliss-Holtz, *Scholarly Inquiry for Nursing Practice: An International Journal*, 5(2), 117. © 1991 by Springer Publishing Company. New York: Springer Publishing Company, Inc., New York 10012. Used by permission.

Mechanisms of Heat Loss. Heat loss in the newborn occurs through four processes: (Figure 4)

• Evaporation — conversion of moisture from the skin and respiratory tract to vapor

• Convection — from the body surface to the surrounding air

• Conduction — from the body surface to a solid surface that is in direct contact

• Radiation — from the body to a cool, solid object not in direct contact with the body

Examples of each mechanism in the newborn are illustrated in Figure 4. Appropriate nursing interventions are included in Table 6.

Heat loss from evaporation in a term newborn is greatest at delivery and during bathing. A wet newborn at birth loses heat with a resultant drop in skin temperature at a rate of 0.3° C/min (0.5° F/min) and rectal temperature by 0.1° C/min (0.2° F/min). This is equivalent to a temperature loss of 3° C (5° F) over 10 minutes (Blackburn & Loper, 1992; Sinclair, 1976). Evaporative losses can be minimized by thoroughly drying the newborn at birth and immediately following a bath, warming soaks and solutions, and warming and humidifying oxygen (see Table 6).

Heat transfer by convection occurs when heat is exchanged between the newborn and the environment by movement of air around the infant. Factors that influence the transfer of heat include: air flow velocity and turbulence, the temperature gradient between the infant's skin and the surrounding air, the amount of subcutaneous tissue, and the amount of exposed skin surface area (Thomas, 1994). Airflow velocity in a closed incubator is fairly consistent, but opening portholes or side panels alters air flow and creates turbulence. Convective losses can be minimized by placing newborns away from drafts; by clothing, swaddling, and using caps for newborns in open cribs; and maintaining the side walls in the up position for a newborn on a radiant warmer bed (see Table 6). The use of warm, humid-

Figure 4. Methods of Heat Loss

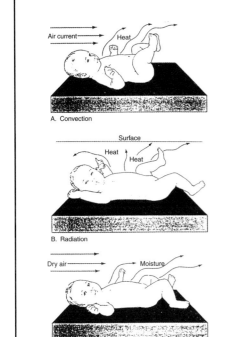

A. Convection

B. Radiation

C. Evaporation

D. Conduction

Note. From *Essentials of Maternal-Newborn Nursing* (3rd ed.) by P. W. Ladewig, M. L. London, and S. B. Olds, 1994, 550. © 1994 by Addison-Wesley Nursing. Redwood City, CA: Addison-Wesley Nursing. Reprinted by permission.

...a constellation of clinical signs directs the process of diagnosis.

ified oxygen also minimizes heat loss and cold stress. Cool, dry oxygen blown across the face stimulates skin thermal receptors, leading to initiation of BAT metabolism (Blackburn & Loper, 1992).

Conductive heat exchange occurs when the neonate comes into direct contact with an object that is cooler or warmer, such as radiograph plates and scales, or warming pads. The larger the surface area in contact with the object, the greater the heat flux. Conductive loss can be minimized by prewarming mattresses, wrapping X-ray plates with warmed blankets, and covering the scale with a warm blanket prior to weighing the newborn (see Table 6). Use of warming pads must be carefully monitored to prevent overheating and thermal burns.

Radiation occurs when heat is exchanged between the body surface to a warmer or cooler surface not in direct contact with the body. Radiation is a movement of heat through air or through a vacuum and is the basis for radiant warmers. Other examples include sunlight coming through an incubator wall or body heat being transferred to a cold wall or window. Radiant heat loss can be minimized by placing infants away from cool exterior walls and windows. Incubators should not be exposed to sunlight, because the plexiglass transmits nearly 100% of the sun's short-wave radiation, which heats the infant. Conversely, none of the infant's long-wave radiation is transmitted back through the plexiglass, so the infant retains excessive heat. In addition, the neonatal nurse must ensure that the newborn is not being overheated when devices such as heat lamps or phototherapy units are being used (see Table 6).

Nursing Assessment. Term infants at increased risk for problems with thermoregulation are presented in Table 7. Newborns who are depressed at birth are particularly at risk for cold stress, which can contribute to metabolic acidosis, increased oxygen demand, hypoxemia and hypoglycemia (Thomas, 1994).

Essential elements of neonatal nursing practice in relation to thermoregulation include:

- Recognition of infants at risk for hypothermia and cold stress and monitoring of all infants for clinical signs

- Monitoring of body temperature and interpreting results

- Initiation of interventions to minimize heat loss for the newborn and prevent cold stress

- Correct use of radiant warmers and incubators in the care of newborns.

Clinical signs and symptoms of cold stress may be subtle and vague and not specific to a diagnosis of cold stress. Cold stress can directly cause observable clinical signs or it may exacerbate other underlying pathology. For example, cool, mottled skin may be a sign of poor perfusion secondary to cardiorespiratory dysfunction and not a response to cold. However, a constellation of clinical signs directs the process of diagnosis. It is therefore important for the neonatal nurse to conduct a thorough systems-based assessment and to consider cold stress as one potential diagnosis. The main physiologic responses to hypothermia and possible clinical signs observable in newborns include:

Table 7. Term Infants at Risk for Problems in Thermoregulation

Infant Category	Basis for Risk
Infants with neurologic problems	Alteration in hypothalamic control
Infants with endocrine problems	Impaired BAT metabolism due to inadequate catecholamine and/or hormones Decreased substrate for energy
Hypoglycemic infants	Decreased metabolic response to cold stress Inability to increase oxygen consumption or minute ventilation further
Infants with cardiorespiratory problems	Inability to increase metabolic rate and reduce metabolic response to cold Impaired BAT metabolism due to hypoxemia Inadequate caloric intake to meet metabolic demands Increased risk of metabolic acidosis Increased temperature losses through evaporation from the lungs
Infants with congenital anomalies such as meningomyelocele, omphalocele, gastroschisis	Increased surface area for heat loss Increased evaporative losses
Small-for-gestational-age infants	Decreased subcutaneous fat insulation Increased surface area for body weight
Sedated infants or maternal intrapartal analgesia	Higher basal metabolic rate and energy demands Limited physical activity to generate heat Maternal diazepam or meperidine associated with decreased newborn temperature

Note. Adapted from "Thermoregulation" by S. T. Blackburn and D. L. Loper. In S. T. Blackburn and D. L. Loper (Eds.), *Maternal, Fetal, and Neonatal Physiology: A Clinical Perspective*, 1992, 691. © 1992 by W. B. Saunders. Adapted by permission.

- Peripheral vasoconstriction. Clinical signs: skin cool, mottled, pale, acrocyanosis, decrease in skin temperature.

- Increased metabolism. Clinical signs: restlessness, crying, increased activity, hypoglycemia, rise in axillary temperature as a result of BAT metabolism.

- Increased oxygen consumption. Clinical signs: tachypnea, grunting, lethargy.

Body Temperature Measurement.
Body temperature in the term newborn is commonly measured via rectal, axillary and skin routes. Rectal temperature approximates core temperature and was traditionally the method of choice for the initial newborn temperature to document both core temperature and rectal patency. Routine use of rectal temperature measurement has declined due to risk of rectal perforation and bradycardia secondary to neurologic stimulation (Blackburn & Loper, 1992; Bliss-Holtz, 1989; Brueggemeyer, 1993). In addition, core temperature is not a sensitive measure of thermal stability. Core temperature is maintained by BAT metabolism and does not change until the infant has lost the ability to produce heat (Darnall, 1987; Dodman, 1987; LeBlanc, 1992).

Axillary temperature measurement is not invasive; however, the axillary fossa contains BAT, which can cause an elevation in axillary temperature when nonshivering thermogenesis is activated (Bliss-Holtz, 1989, 1991, 1993; Merenstein & Gardner, 1993). This effect on axillary temperature particularly affects term newborns because sufficient axillary BAT for significant heat production is present after 34 weeks gestation (Bliss-Holtz, 1995). Figure 5 shows a comparison of skin,

axillary and rectal temperature measurements in a cool infant, with the axillary temperature rising even as the rectal temperature falls. In light of the effects of BAT metabolism on core and axillary temperatures, perhaps one site of body temperature measurement is inadequate to assess a newborn for cold stress (Bliss-Holtz, 1991).

There is no consensus in the literature regarding the optimal method for obtaining an accurate axillary temperature using a glass mercury thermometer. Published studies on term newborns report optimal axillary temperatures reached by the majority of infants by five minutes in two studies (Haddock, Vincent, & Merrow, 1986; Mayfield, Bhatia, Nakamura, Rios, & Bell, 1984); by five and one-half minutes in one study (Bliss-Holtz, 1989); and 11 minutes in two studies (Kunnel, O'Brien, Munro, & Medoff-Cooper, 1988; Stephan & Sexton, 1987). Stephan and Sexton (1987) reported the greatest difference between five minutes and stabilization, 0.17° F, which was not statistically significant. This difference may not be clinically significant in a term, low-risk newborn. In terms of electronic temperature measurement, Hunter (1991) reported a high correlation between axillary electronic and glass mercury temperature recordings. This research evidence lends support to the common practice of using electronic thermometers.

Skin temperature changes occur early in response to heat losses and gains. Presently, skin temperature measurement is not routinely used for term newborns except as servo control when supplemental heat is provided via radiant warmer or incubator. Two studies including full-term infants have incorporated skin-to-mattress temperature measurement (Kunnel, et al., 1988; Mayfield, et al., 1984). The site was found to yield lower readings than

MARCH OF DIMES NURSING MODULE

Figure 5. Temperature Measurement at Various Sites During Cold Stress

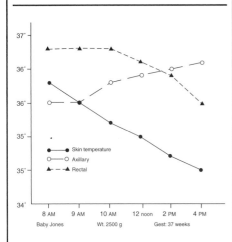

- ● Skin temperature
- ○ Axillary
- ▲ Rectal

8 AM 9 AM 10 AM 12 noon 2 PM 4 PM
Baby Jones   Wt. 2500 g   Gest: 37 weeks

In an environment that is less than thermal neutral, cold stress begins as skin temperature decreases (9 am) because of vasoconstriction of skin. 10 am: Axillary temperature increases as infant burns brown fat to keep warm: rectal temperature is unchanged, since core temperature is maintained. Noon: Infant is still cold stressed (skin temperature is down); axillary temperature is up as infant continues to compensate (burns brown fat); rectal temperature is still in normal range. 2 pm to 4 pm: Skin temperature reflects severe cold stress; axilla is warm but baby is cold; rectal (core temperature) falls as body decompensates — severe cold stress.

Note. From *Handbook of Neonatal Intensive Care* (2nd ed.) by G. B. Merenstein and S. L. Gardner, (1989). © 1989 by C. V. Mosby. Reprinted by permission.

axillary and rectal sites and norms have not been established.

Two additional sites for temperature measurement in the newborn are inguinal/femoral and tympanic membrane. Inguinal/femoral site temperature measurement has been tested in two studies and may hold future promise as an alternative site for monitoring body temperature that is not influenced by BAT (Bliss-Holtz, 1989; Kunnel, et al., 1988). Norms for the inguinal site have not been determined. Research on infrared tympanic thermometry for neonatal temperature assessment has found poor correlations between axillary and tympanic measurement (Weiss, 1991), more variation between tympanic and axillary and between tympanic and rectal than between axillary and rectal readings (Weiss, Poeltler, & Gocka, 1994), and variation of more than 0.6° F from rectal temperatures measured by glass mercury thermometers (Yetman, Coody, West, Montgomery, & Brown, 1993). Clinical use of tympanic membrane thermometry cannot yet be recommended for newborns.

Nursing Assessment of Body Temperature. Presently axillary temperature measurement is the preferred method of newborn temperature assessment. For glass mercury thermometers, five minutes is an appropriate placement time to reach optimum temperature. The neonatal nurse should keep in mind the possible effects of BAT metabolism on the axillary temperature and assess the newborn for other signs of thermal stability.

External Heat Sources. A term newborn who is unable to achieve or maintain body temperature requires supplemental external heat to prevent complications from cold stress. Supplemental heat is provided through the use of a convective incubator or a radiant warmer. An incubator provides heat by circulating warm air (convection) and minimizes heat loss by providing a closed, controlled environment. Temperature control within the incubator is accomplished via air or skin servo control or manual control. With servo control, air or skin temperature is electronically monitored and used to control heater output. The desired skin temperature is 36° C to 36.5° C (Glatzl-Hawlik & Bell, 1992).

Appropriate sites for placement of skin temperature probes include the skin surface over the liver and between the umbilicus and pubis (Blackburn & Loper, 1992). The infant can become hyperthermic if the skin probe becomes detached. Heater output must be monitored with servo control to track the amount of supplemental heat the infant is requiring, as an increasing need for supplemental support could be an early indication of infection. Body temperature must be closely monitored when the manual heater control is used. The incubator must be preheated before use, placed away from direct sunlight to prevent radiant heat gain and hyperthermia, and away from cool drafts that cool the walls of the incubator and increase radiant heat loss from the infant to the walls of the incubator. Heat is lost from the incubator when portholes are opened.

Nursing Management of Infant in Incubator

- Incubator air temperature is adjusted based on neonatal age and weight; use guidelines as beginning set point. (See Table 8.)

- Portholes and doors must be kept closed unless providing care.

- The newborn's temperature must be monitored to determine temperature stability.

- The newborn may be naked or dressed while in the incubator.

- If dressed while in the incubator, air temperature should be frequently monitored; the isolette should be set on air control.

- If naked, skin temperature should be monitored using a skin probe, and the incubator should be set on skin control.

Table 8.
Neutral Thermal Environment Temperatures for Newborns with Birthweights Over 2500 gms and Greater Than 36 Weeks Gestation

Age	Range of Temperature (°C)
0-6 hours	32.0-33.8
6-12 hours	31.4-33.8
12-24 hours	31.0-33.7
24-36 hours	30.7-33.5
36-48 hours	30.5-33.3
48-72 hours	30.1-33.2
72-96 hours	29.8-32.8

Note. Adapted from *Care of the High-Risk Neonate* (4th ed.) by M. H. Klaus and A. A. Fanaroff, 1993, 121. © 1993 by W. B. Saunders. Reprinted by permission.

Radiant warmers provide a powerful radiant heat source and maintain the newborn's temperature through a servo control mechanism. The radiant heat must be able to reach the infant's skin; therefore, the use of hats and clothing are inappropriate for infants under radiant warmers. Under the radiant warmer, the skin probe should be covered with a reflective patch to prevent direct heating of the probe and falsely high skin temperature readings. Even with the use of a reflective patch, however, the skin probe may indicate a temperature that is higher than the rest of the infant's body. This error occurs because the skin probe is insulated by the tape or adhesive patch attaching it to the skin and evaporative losses are reduced (Blackburn & Loper, 1992). An infant may therefore require a higher setting for the desired skin temperature in order to maintain overall body temperature. An infant can quickly become hyperthermic under a radiant warmer if the skin probe detaches or if the manual setting is used.

Nursing Management of Newborn Under Radiant Warmer

- Use servo control setting with skin probe; check probe routinely for detachment.
- Keep side walls in up position to minimize convective heat loss.
- Monitor infant body temperature.
- Do not use head covering or clothing.

Rewarming of a hypothermic newborn requires frequent and careful monitoring of the infant's response. Radiant warmers permit more rapid warming than incubators. Complications of rapid rewarming include heat-induced apnea and decreased blood pressure and shock secondary to rapid vasodilation (Blackburn & Loper, 1992; Glatzl-

Hawlik & Bell, 1992). Slow rewarming risks further complications from the effects of cold stress.

Hyperthermia. The newborn is also at risk for hyperthermia (>37.5° C), primarily secondary to overheating and less commonly to hypermetabolism (Blackburn & Loper, 1992). Physiologic consequences of hyperthermia and possible clinical signs in the term newborn are as follows:

- Peripheral vasodilation. Clinical signs: flushed, warm extremities; decreased blood pressure; sweating; skin temperature higher than core temperature

- Increased metabolism. Clinical signs: increased activity; irritability

- Increased oxygen consumption. Clinical signs: increased respiratory rate; increased heart rate.

Body temperature must be monitored frequently as the infant is allowed to cool.

Thermoregulation is vital to the newborn infant and virtually entirely managed by nursing. Neonatal nurses must understand mechanisms of heat losses and gains, be knowledgeable regarding assessments and interventions, and correctly interpret body temperature measurements in order to facilitate thermal stability and homeostasis in the newborn.

Assessment of Gestational Age

Prior to 1960, birthweight was the only criterion used to determine a newborn's maturity. Consequently, an infant whose birthweight was greater than 2500 grams (5 lbs., 5 oz.) was considered term. Newborn size, however, is affected by conditions that accelerate or retard fetal growth, resulting in discrepancies between growth and maturity. For example,

Rewarming of a hypothermic newborn requires frequent and careful monitoring of the infant's response.

infants of diabetic mothers may be born prematurely but larger than a term infant, and conversely, when uteroplacental insufficiency is present, an infant may be born at term but be small. Accurate assessment of gestational age now incorporates size and maturity, facilitating identification of infants at risk, anticipation of clinical problems and planning of care (see Figure 6).

Definitions. Gestational age is defined as the number of weeks from the first day of the mother's last normal menstrual period to the time of birth. Commonly accepted definitions of preterm, term and postterm newborns are as follows: a preterm infant is born before the completion of the 37th week of gestation; a term newborn is born between the beginning of the 38th week and the completion of

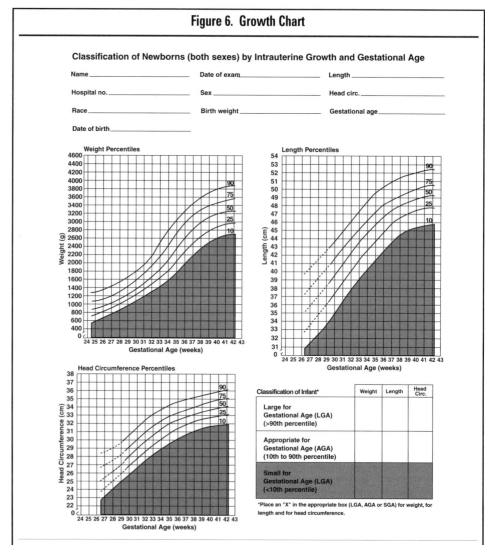

Figure 6. Growth Chart

Classification of Newborns (both sexes) by Intrauterine Growth and Gestational Age

Note. From Ross Laboratories publication: 10-91; (0.05) A-58560, constructed from Battaglia F.C., & Lubchenco, L.O. (1967). A practical classification of newborn infants by weight and gestational age. Journal of Pediatrics, 71, 159-163, and Lubchenco, L.O., Hansman, C., & Boyd, E. (1966). Intrauterine growth in length and head circumference as estimated from live births at gestational ages from 26 to 42 weeks. Pediatrics 37, 403-408. Reprinted by permission of Ross Laboratories, The American Academy of Pediatrics, Mosby-Year Book, F.C. Battaglia, and L.O. Lubchenko.

the 41st week; and any infant born after the start of the 42nd week of pregnancy is considered postterm.

Estimating Gestational Age. Gestational age is estimated by the calculation of dates based on the mother's last menstrual period (LMP), evaluation of obstetrical indicators and neonatal examination. Calculation based on the LMP can be difficult when the exact date of the LMP is not known, when periods have been irregular, or when postconceptional bleeding is confused with menstruation. The expected accuracy and reliability of dating based on the last normal menstrual period is ± 14.6 days, a total range of four weeks (Attico, Meyer, Bodin, & Dickman, 1990). Accuracy and reliability of various obstetrical methods for determining gestational age range from ± seven to 10 days for an ultrasound prior to 14 weeks gestation, to ± three weeks for detection of fetal heart tones by Doppler between nine and 12 weeks (Attico, et al., 1990). Estimation of gestational age of the newborn is based on a combination of the physical exam and assessment of neurological capabilities. The neurologic responses are based on expected progression of neuromuscular maturation, which consists of replacement of extensor tone by flexor tone in a caudocephalad (tail-to-head) progression (Hill, 1992; Ladewig, et al., 1994). The Dubowitz Assessment of Gestational Age, published in 1970 by Dubowitz, Dubowitz, and Goldberg, consists of 11 external physical characteristics and 10 neurologic signs.

The external physical signs include skin characteristics, plantar creases, nipple and breast development, ear development and formation, and appearance of the genitalia. Neurologic signs include resting posture, square window, ankle dorsiflexion, arm and leg recoil, popliteal angle, heel to ear, scarf sign, head lag and ventral suspension. Ballard and his colleagues devised a simplified Maturational Score based on the Dubowitz, using six neuromuscular and six physical criteria that could be performed within two to four minutes with comparable reliability to the Dubowitz (Ballard, Novak, & Driver, 1979) (see Figures 7-13 for illustrations; see Figure 14 for assignment of Ballard Score).

Overall accuracy of the Dubowitz and Ballard examinations are expected to be accurate to within ± 2 weeks (Alexander & Allen, 1996). A comparison of the Ballard, LMP, and ultrasound assessments found close agreement among the measures at 40 weeks, but the Ballard score tended to overestimate gestational age for preterm and underestimate for postterm infants (Alexander, de Caunes, Hulsey, Tompkins, & Allen, 1992). A revised or New Ballard Score (Ballard, Khoury, Wedig, Wang, Ellers-Walsman, & Lipp, 1991) has been developed that includes signs for the extremely premature infant and can be used for infants from 20 to 44 weeks gestation (Figure 14). This tool is the focus in this module.

Estimation of gestational age of the newborn is based on a combination of the physical exam and assessment of neurological capabilities.

Table 9. Instructions for Use of the Ballard Gestational Age Assessment Tool

Neuromuscular Maturity

Posture is the position the baby naturally assumes when lying quietly on his back. A very premature infant will lie with arms and legs extended in whatever posture he is placed. As intrauterine development progresses, the fetus is capable of more and more flexion. When born at term, an infant lies with his arms flexed to his chest, his hands fisted, and his legs flexed towards his abdomen (see Figure 8).

Square window (wrist) is the angle achieved when the infant's palm is flexed toward his forearm. A premature infant's wrist exhibits poor flexion and makes a 90-degree angle with the arm. An extremely immature infant has no flexor tone and can-not achieve even 90-degree flexion. A term infant's wrist will flex completely against the forearm. This can also be done with the ankle, but ankle flexion was excluded from the Ballard tool because it duplicates the wrist flexion and may not be possible or accurate in babies with intrauterine posi-tional effects (see Figure 9).

Arm recoil is elicited by first flexing the arms at the elbows to the chest, then fully extending them and releasing. Term infants will resist extension and briskly return their arms to the flexed position. Very preterm infants will not resist exten-sion and respond with weak and delayed flexion in a small arc. The flexion angle of the elbow is estimated (see Figure 10).

Popliteal angle is assessed with the infant lying supine. Keeping his pelvis flat, flex his thigh to his abdomen and hold it there while extending his leg at the knee. The angle at the knee is estimated (see Figure 11). The preterm infant will achieve greater extension.

Scarf sign is elicited by moving the baby's arm across his chest as far toward the opposite shoulder as possible while he is lying supine (Figure 12). The term infant's elbow will not cross midline, but it will be possible to bring the preterm infant's elbow much farther toward the opposite shoulder.

Heel to ear is similar to popliteal angle, but the knee and thigh are not held in place. The baby's foot is drawn as near to the head or ear as possible. Scoring is based on the distance from heel to head. The premature baby will be able to get his foot close to his head (see Figure 13).

Physical Maturity

Skin is assessed for thickness, transparency and texture. Premature skin is thin, with visible vessels, and smooth. Extremely preterm infants have sticky, transparent skin. A term infant's skin is thick, veins are difficult to see and the texture may be flaky.

Lanugo is the fine hair seen over the back of premature babies by 24 weeks. It begins to thin over the lower back first and disappears last over the shoulders.

Plantar creases are the deep folds and creases seen over the bottom of the foot. One or two appear over the pad of the foot at approximately 32 weeks. At 36 weeks, the creases cover the anterior two-thirds of the foot. At term, they cover the whole foot (see Figure 7). At very early gestation, the length of the sole is measured. For extremely immature infants, this item was expanded to include foot length mea-sured from the tip of the great toe to the back of the heel.

Breast tissue is examined for visibility of nipple and areola and size of bud when grasped between thumb and forefinger. The very premature infant will not have visible nipples or are-ola. These become more defined and then raised by 34 weeks, with a small bud appearing at 36 weeks and growing to 5-10 mm by term (see Figure 7).

Ear formation includes the development of cartilage and the curving of the pinnae. Lack of cartilage in earlier gesta-tion results in the ear folding easily and retaining this fold. As gestation progresses, soft cartilage can be felt with increasing resistance to folding and increasing recoil. The pinnae are flat in very preterm infants. Incurving proceeds from the top down toward the lobes as gestation advances (see Figure 7).

Eyes in the extremely immature infant are examined, and the degree of eyelid fusion is assessed with gentle traction.

Genitalia are virtually indistinguishable at 20 weeks. In males, the testes are in the inguinal canal around 28 weeks, and rugae are beginning to be visible. By 36 weeks, the testes are in the upper scrotum, and rugae cover the anterior por-tion of the scrotum. At term, rugae cover the scrotum, and at postterm the testes are pendulous. In females, the clitoris is initially prominent and the labia minora are flat. By 36 weeks, the labia majora are larger and the clitoris is nearly covered (see Figure 7).

Note. Adapted from "Gestational Age Assessment" by V. Dodd, *Neonatal Network*, 1996, 15(1), 27-36. Adapted by permission.

Figure 7. Physical Assessment

An illustrated guide to gestational age

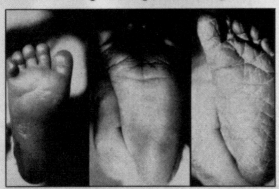

The feet are smooth (left) through the 35th week when creases start appearing on the upper third (center); by term they are creased from top to bottom (right).

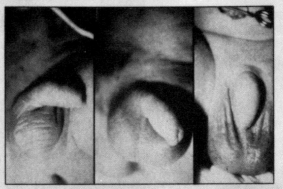

The testes start descending at about 36 weeks (left). They remain in the upper scrotum for a few weeks (center) and are palpable in the lower scrotum at term (right).

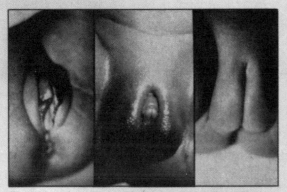

The labia are small, revealing a prominent clitoris (left), before 35 weeks. They begin to grow thereafter (center) and by term, they cover the clitoris completely (right).

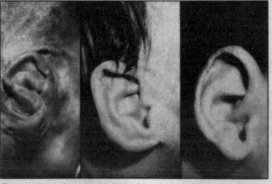

Ear cartilage is essentially lacking before 35 weeks (left) but by 38 weeks there's enough to allow the pinna to open up when folded (center). The full-term infant's ear springs back almost as fast as an adult's (right).

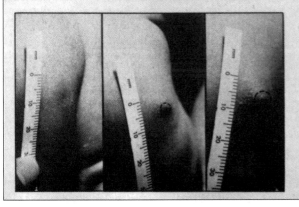

Only the areola is visible in the earlier stages of gestation (left) but between 36 and 38 weeks you can feel a 1- to 2-mm nodule of breast tissue (center). And the term infant will have 7 to 10 mm of breast tissue (right).

Note. From "Determining Gestational Age" By A.W. Brann, *Emergency Medicine*, October 1977, 9(10), 51-64. © 1977 by Fisher Medical Publications. Reprinted by permission.

Figure 8. Posture Scoring

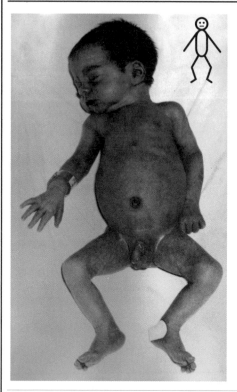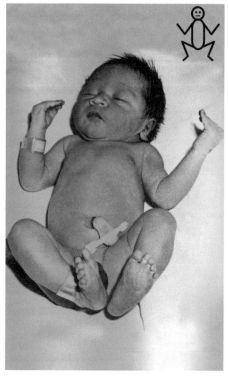

Note. From *Gestational Age of the Newborn* by L. M. S. Dubowitz and V. Dubowitz, 1977, 62, 64. © 1977 by Addison-Wesley. Reprinted by permission.

Figure 9. Square Window Scoring

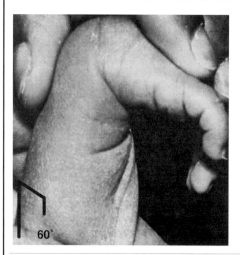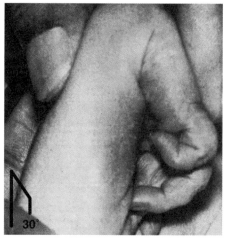

Note. From *Gestational Age of the Newborn* by L. M. S. Dubowitz and V. Dubowitz, 1977, 66, 67. © 1977 by Addison-Wesley. Reprinted by permission.

Figure 10. Demonstration of Method for Eliciting Arm Recoil

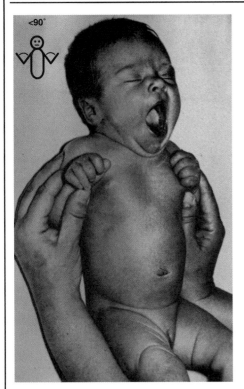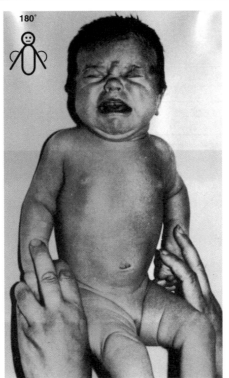

Note. From *Gestational Age of the Newborn* by L. M. S. Dubowitz and V. Dubowitz, 1977, 66, 67. © 1977 by Addison-Wesley. Reprinted by permission.

Figure 11. Popliteal Angle Scoring

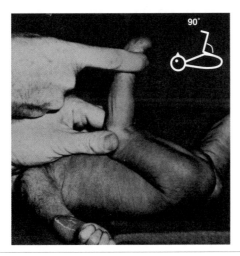

Note. From *Gestational Age of the Newborn* by L. M. S. Dubowitz and V. Dubowitz, 1977, 66, 67. © 1977 by Addison-Wesley. Reprinted by permission.

Figure 12. Scarf Sign Scoring

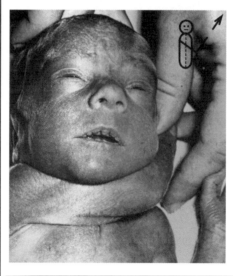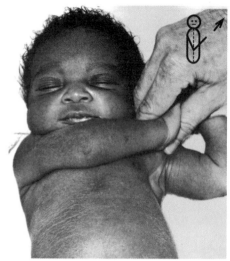

Note. From *Gestational Age of the Newborn* by L. M. S. Dubowitz and V. Dubowitz, 1977, 66, 67. © 1977 by Addison-Wesley. Reprinted by permission.

Figure 13. Heel to Ear Scoring

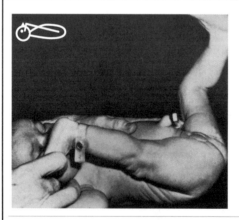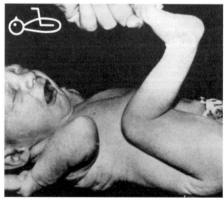

Note. From *Gestational Age of the Newborn* by L. M. S. Dubowitz and V. Dubowitz, 1977, 66, 67. © 1977 by Addison-Wesley. Reprinted by permission.

Figure 14. New Ballard Score

Neuromuscular Maturity

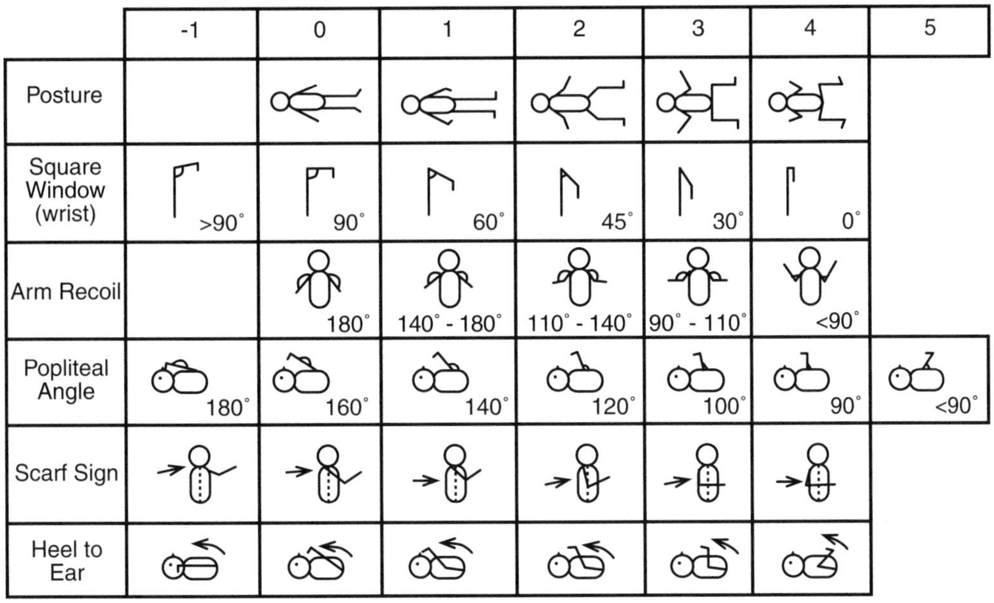

	-1	0	1	2	3	4	5
Posture							
Square Window (wrist)	>90°	90°	60°	45°	30°	0°	
Arm Recoil		180°	140° - 180°	110° - 140°	90° - 110°	<90°	
Popliteal Angle	180°	160°	140°	120°	100°	90°	<90°
Scarf Sign							
Heel to Ear							

Physical Maturity

Skin	sticky friable transparent	gelatinous red, translucent	smooth pink visible veins	superficial peeling &/or rash few veins	cracking pale areas rare veins	parchment deep cracking no vessels	leathery cracked wrinkled
Lanugo	none	sparse	abundant	thinning	bald areas	mostly bald	
Plantar Surface	heel-toe 40-50 mm:-1 < 40 mm:-2	>50mm no crease	faint red marks	anterior transverse crease only	creases ant. 2/3	creases over entire sole	
Breast	imperceptible	barely perceptible	flat areola no bud	slipped areola 1-2mm bud	raised areola 3-4mm bud	full areola 5-10mm bud	
Eye/Ear	lids fused loosely:-1 tightly:-2	lids open pinna flat stays folded	sl. curved pinna; soft; slow recoil	well-curved pinna: soft but ready recoil	formed & firm instant recoil	thick cartillage ear stiff	
Genitals male	scrotum flat, smooth	scrotum empty faint rugae	testes in upper canal rare rugae	testes descending few rugae	testes down good rugae	testes pendulous deep rugae	
Genitals female	clitoris prominent labia flat	prominent clitoris small labia minora	prominent clitoris enlarging minora	majora & minora equally prominent	majora large minora small	majora cover clitoris & minora	

Maturity Rating

score	weeks
-10	20
-5	22
-0	24
5	26
10	28
15	30
20	32
25	34
30	36
35	38
40	40
45	42
50	44

Note. From "New Ballard Score, Expanded to Include Extremely Premature Infants" by J. L. Ballard, J. C. Khoury, K. Wedig, L. Wang, B.L. Eilers-Walsman, & R. Lipp. *Journal of Pediatrics*, 119(3), 418. © 1991 by Mosby Year-Book, Inc. Reprinted by permission.

Although optimal timing of the examination is not specific, the preferred infant state is one of quiet alertness, where the infant is responsive but not agitated (Blackburn, 1990).

Timing of the Examination. There is no consensus regarding the optimal timing for gestational age examination. Dubowitz and associates performed multiple examinations on 70 newborns and reported no significant difference in reliability between assessments performed during the first 24 hours of life and those conducted after 24 hours up to five days of age (Dubowitz, et al., 1970). Ballard and colleagues (1979) reported reliability for the original Ballard Maturational Score to be greatest when performed on the newborn between 30 and 42 hours of age. Recommendations for performing the New Ballard Score are within the first 12 hours of life for infants of less than 26 weeks gestation, and within the first 96 hours of life for other infants (Ballard, et al., 1991). Concern regarding timing of the exam centers on changes in the newborn's tone and reflexes during the first days of life. Reliability of neuromuscular maturity assessment is greater after 30 hours of age for infants who are beyond 26 weeks gestation (Ballard, et al., 1991). Physical maturity may be more accurately assessed during the first several hours after birth, however, and the gestational age examination is sometimes performed with other admission assessments. When this is the practice, the neuromuscular maturity assessment may need to be repeated, particularly if findings from the first exam differ from obstetrical dating or if the infant's condition is complicated by central nervous system depression during the early transitional period (AAP/ACOG, Guidelines for Perinatal Care, 1992; Trotter, 1993). Although optimal timing of the examination is not specific, the preferred infant state is one of quiet alertness, where the infant is responsive but not agitated (Blackburn, 1990).

Prior to performing the examination, the neonatal nurse should note the age of the newborn in hours; the newborn's weight, length and occipital-frontal head circumference (OFC); gestational age as estimated from date of LMP and obstetrical indicators; the newborn's immediate transition to extrauterine life; Apgar scores, resuscitative efforts at delivery, signs of central nervous system depression; and maternal and infant risk factors.

Maintenance of thermal stability during the examination is imperative. The gestational age examination can be integrated with a complete physical examination by an experienced examiner.

Instructions for use of the Ballard Gestational Age Assessment Tool are in Table 9. A score is assigned for each item. If a sign falls between the scoring options, a half score may be assigned (Dodd, 1996). After assessing and scoring all 12 items, a total score is calculated and compared to the maturity rating table to estimate the infant's gestational age in weeks. For example, a score of 37 would correspond to a gestational age between 38 and 40 weeks.

Infant Classification. Following determination of infant maturity by gestational age exam, the infant's length, weight, and OFC are plotted on intrauterine growth curves as shown in Figures 6 and 15. Growth curves provide measures of intrauterine growth in percentiles for each week of gestation. Infants who are above the 90th percentile are termed Large for Gestational Age (LGA), infants below the 10th percentile are Small for Gestational Age (SGA), and infants between the 10th and 90th percentiles are considered Appropriate for Gestational Age (AGA). For example, a newborn weighing 3600 gm at 40 weeks is term AGA but an infant weighing 3600 gm at 37 weeks is term LGA on this growth curve (Figure 15). Within the first 24 hours, the OFC may be affected by molding or caput succedaneum (scalp edema). Term newborns can therefore be classified as AGA, SGA or LGA. Term newborns who are AGA have lower mortality (Figure 15) and morbidity (Figure 16) rates than those who are SGA or LGA (Battaglia & Lubchenco, 1967).

Several intrauterine growth curves have been developed based on differ-ent populations. Two commonly used curves are the Oregon and Denver curves. The Oregon curves were normed on 40,000 live, singleton infants born at sea level between 1959 and 1966 to Caucasian women who were cared for by private physicians (Babson, Behrman, & Lessel, 1970). The Colorado curves (Figure 15) were based on 4,700 newborns born to med-ically indigent white (55%), Hispanic (30%) and black (15%) mothers at an altitude of 5,280 feet (Lubchenco, Searles, & Brazie, 1972). Infants born at high altitude are somewhat smaller

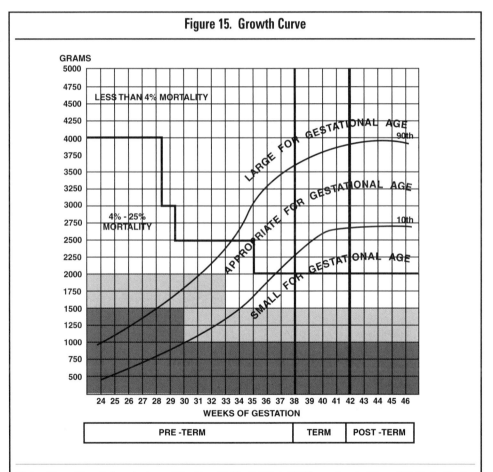

Figure 15. Growth Curve

Note. From Ross Laboratories publication: 10-91; (0.05) A-58560 constructed from F.C. Battaglia & L.O. Lubchenco, 1967. "A Practical Classification of Newborn Infants by Weight and Gestational Age," *Journal of Pediatrics*, 71, 159-163, and L.O. Lubchenco, C. Hansman, & E. Boyd, 1966, "Intrauterine Growth in Length and Head Circumference as Estimated from Live Births at Gestational Ages from 26 to 42 Weeks," *Pediatrics*, 37, 403-408. Reprinted by permission of Ross Laboratories, The American Academy of Pediatrics, and Mosby-Year Book.

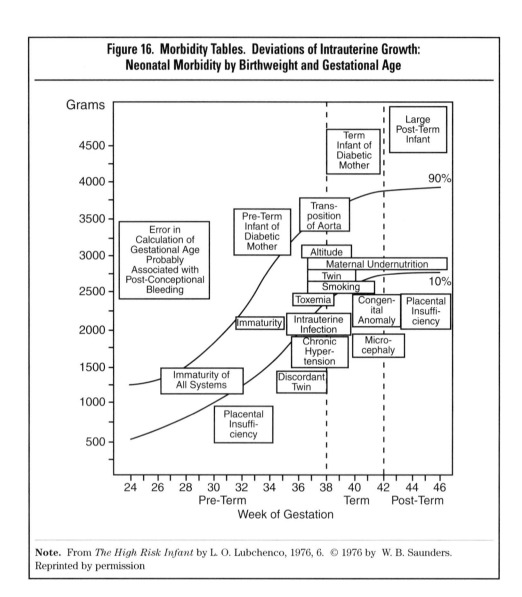

Figure 16. Morbidity Tables. Deviations of Intrauterine Growth: Neonatal Morbidity by Birthweight and Gestational Age

Note. From *The High Risk Infant* by L. O. Lubchenco, 1976, 6. © 1976 by W. B. Saunders. Reprinted by permission

than infants born at sea level and maternal health and nutritional status affect fetal growth rates. The Oregon curves include weight only.

Large for Gestational Age

Large for gestational age is associated with postdates gestation, maternal diabetes with hyperglycemia, maternal obesity, genetically large babies (of large parents), transposition of the great vessels, Beckwith-Wiedemann Syndrome and erythroblastosis fetalis (Dodd, 1996; Trotter, 1993). Genetically large newborns do not have increased

risks related to pathophysiologic processes. Infants of diabetic mothers with poor serum glucose control receive excess glucose via the placenta and respond with hyperinsulinemia. Consequently, these infants are prone to excess body fat and glycogen stores, increased muscle mass and organomegaly, especially heart and liver (Cowett, 1992). LGA infants are at increased risk for prolonged labor, shoulder dystocia, birth injury, postnatal respiratory depression from difficult deliveries, and hypoglycemia (secondary to fetal hyperinsulinism)

(Blackburn, 1990). Types of birth injuries to assess for include: bruising, cephalohematomas, facial nerve palsy, fractured clavicle, and brachial plexus injury. Infants with cephalohematomas are at increased risk for hyperbilirubinemia. Screening blood glucose levels is an important consideration for these infants.

Small for Gestational Age

Maternal factors contributing to the incidence of an SGA birth include poor maternal weight gain during pregnancy, multiparity, chronic maternal disease, multiple gestation and uteroplacental insufficiency (heart disease, renal disease, hypertension, preeclampsia, postterm pregnancy, sickle cell disease, or smoking). Fetal factors include chromosomal abnormalities, malformations in the skeletal system or congenital infections such as cytomegalovirus or rubella (Gunderson, Cantu, Vaello, & Brueggemeyer, 1993). Conditions associated with SGA place such newborns at greater risk for mortality than infants born AGA or LGA. Two types of growth retardation are classified. Symmetrical or nonhead-sparing growth retardation refers to a constant but slower pattern of fetal growth where length, weight and OFC (brain growth) are all reduced. In asymmetrical or head-sparing growth retardation, fetal growth slows and may even stop. Brain growth is preserved over organ and body growth, resulting in OFC being less affected than length measurements and weight affected the most (Sparks & Cetin, 1992). The terms SGA and intrauterine growth retardation (IUGR) are often used synonymously. Intrauterine growth retardation is more accurately used to denote a pathophysiologic process that results in fetal growth restriction, whereas SGA refers categorically to infants who fall below the 10th percentile on a growth curve (Sparks &

Cetin, 1992). IUGR infants are often SGA; however, a fetus who has stopped growing in utero and is delivered before falling below the 10th percentile is correctly termed IUGR, even though not SGA.

SGA newborns are at increased risk for hypoglycemia, secondary to diminished glycogen stores; hypothermia due to decreased subcutaneous tissue; hypoxia during labor and delivery, particularly when growth retardation results from chronic uteroplacental insufficiency; polycythemia and hyperbilirubinemia.

Postterm Newborns

Newborns born after 42 weeks gestation are at risk for uteroplacental insufficiency and postmaturity syndrome. Most infants born postterm are healthy. Some continue to grow and are LGA, while others may appear thin and wasted secondary to utero-placental insufficiency. Approximately 5% show signs of postmaturity syndrome, as a result of uteroplacental insufficiency, with increased risk for mortality. The postmature infant is at risk for hypoglycemia from decreased nutritional support and depleted glycogen stores; meconium release and aspiration secondary to intrauterine hypoxia; polycythemia due to increased red blood cell production in response to hypoxia; neurologic signs and symptoms as a result of hypoxia and asphyxia; and hypothermia due to loss of subcutaneous tissue.

Nursing Management for LGA and SGA Newborns. Nursing management for LGA and SGA newborns involves close monitoring of transition to extrauterine life, to assess for: complications related to hypoxia or asphyxia, physical and gestational age examination for accurate classification and risk assessment, assessment for congenital anomalies, glucose instability and

Recognition of specific states of consciousness enables neonatal nurses to better interpret physiologic and behavioral changes.

consideration of early feedings, assessment for polycythemia and observation for jaundice. In addition, SGA newborns must be monitored for thermal stability, and LGA infants should be closely assessed for birth injuries.

Postnatal determination of gestational age provides direct evidence of newborn maturity and intrauterine growth. It is particularly helpful in situations where late or inadequate prenatal care precludes full obstetrical dating or knowledge regarding LMP is uncertain. Further classification of newborns as SGA, AGA and LGA facilitates appropriate risk assessment and anticipation of complications.

Patterns of Sleep and Activity

A term, nonstressed neonate can be expected to follow a predictable pattern of behavior during the initial hours after birth. The first six to eight hours after birth are referred to as the *transitional period*, a term used by Desmond, Franklin, Valbona, Hill, Plumb, Arnold, and Watts, (1963). During this time the newborn experiences behavioral changes related to sleep/awake states and response to stimuli, as well as variation in physiologic parameters during three periods: an initial period of reactivity immediately after birth, a period of relative inactivity and a second period of reactivity. The sequence of periods is consistent among newborns, but the timing and length of each period varies and is influenced by such factors as maternal medications and length of labor (Lott, 1993). Time periods may also differ from Desmond's observations during the 1960s because of changes in management of labor and delivery, maternal medications and initiation of earlier newborn feedings.

During the *initial period of reactivity* (during approximately the first hour after birth), the newborn is alert, active

and exhibits a strong desire to suck, providing an excellent opportunity for a breastfeeding mother to nurse her infant for the first time. This is also a good time for parent-newborn interaction. Delaying the instillation of prophylactic eye medication until after this period permits the newborn to better respond visually to the parents (Lott, 1993). Physiologically the neonate may be tachypneic (up to 80 breaths/minute), tachycardic (up to 180 beats/minute), and exhibit mild to moderate chest wall retractions, grunting and flaring. Acrocyanosis is expected during this time but central cyanosis is not normal. Other signs of risk include apnea greater than 15 seconds, asymmetrical chest wall movement, unequal breath sounds, excessive salivation and mucous, and lethargy.

Two to three hours after birth, responsiveness to surroundings gradually decreases until the neonate falls asleep for a period lasting anywhere from a few minutes to several hours. During this time, the *period of relative inactivity*, the newborn will show little interest in external stimuli and will arouse only with difficulty. Respiratory rate may increase during sleep with heart rate ranging from 120-140 beats/minute.

The *second period of reactivity*, lasting from four to six hours, begins when the newborn awakens from this first sleep. The infant is alert and responsive again, and heart and respiratory rates increase. The first urine and meconium stool are often passed during this period. Heart and respiratory rates stabilize and become more regular as this period ends.

Infant State Assessment

Evaluation of newborn behavior incorporates assessment of state of consciousness, reactions to stimulation, and the newborn's ability to move from one state to another (Brazelton, 1984; Thoman, 1990). Newborn behavior and physiological parameters are affected by state of consciousness. A healthy term newborn demonstrates an individual and organized pattern of distinct states of consciousness over time. The state behavior pattern of organization is an indicator of general well-being and central nervous system integrity, as well as a measure of the newborn's response to external stimuli. Recognition of specific states of consciousness enables neonatal nurses to better interpret physiologic and behavioral changes. Assessment of infant state is therefore an appropriate and important aspect of neonatal care (Kaminski & Hall, 1996; Brazelton, 1984).

Infants who experience perinatal complications have been found to display different state patterns compared to healthy full-term newborns (Holditch-Davis, 1993). SGA term newborns demonstrate more disorganized sleep and poorer responsiveness during alertness (Holditch-Davis, 1993).

Brazelton's neonatal behavioral assessment scale (NBAS) is a state scoring system consisting of a total of six states, two sleep and four awake states (Brazelton, 1984). These include deep sleep, light sleep, drowsy, quiet alert, active alert and crying. Table 10 provides the characteristics of each state and implications for caregiving. The quiet alert state is the optimal state for feeding and for parent-infant interactions (Holditch-Davis, 1993). It is also the best state during which to perform a gestational age exam.

The Brazelton assessment and others (Thoman, 1990) provide further information regarding the infant's ability to engage a primary caregiver's attention through states of consciousness. Performance of the Brazelton assessment in the mother's presence allows the examiner to identify individual newborn characteristics and to educate parents regarding infant state.

Table 10. Infant State Chart (Sleep and Awake States)

STATE is a group of characteristics that regularly occur together: body activity, eye movements, facial movements, breathing pattern and level of response to external stimuli (e.g., handling) and internal stimuli (e.g., hunger).

Characteristics of State

Sleep States	Body Activity	Eye Movements	Facial Movements	Breathing Pattern	Level of Response	Implications for Caregiving
Deep Sleep	Nearly still, except for occasional startle or twitch.	None.	Without facial movements, except for occasional sucking movements at regular intervals.	Smooth and regular.	Threshold to stimuli is very high so that only very intense and disturbing stimuli will arouse infants.	Caregivers trying to feed infants in deep sleep will probably find the experience frustrating. Infants will be unresponsive even if caregivers use disturbing stimuli (flicking feet) to arouse infants. Infants may only arouse briefly and then become unresponsive as they return to deep sleep. If caregivers wait until infants move to a higher, more responsive state, feeding or caregiving will be much more pleasant.
Light Sleep	Some body movements.	Rapid eye movements (Rem), fluttering of eyes beneath closed eyelids.	May smile and make brief fussy or crying sounds.	Irregular.	More responsive to internal and external stimuli. When these stimuli occur infants may remain in light sleep, return to deep sleep or arouse to drowsy.	Light sleep makes up the highest proportion of newborn sleep and usually precedes wakening. Due to brief fussy or crying sounds made during this state, caregivers who are not aware that these sounds occur normally may think it is time for feeding and may try to feed infants before they are ready to eat.
Drowsy	Activity level variable, with mild startles interspersed from time to time. Movements usually smooth.	Eyes open and close occasionally, are heavy-lidded with dull, glazed appearance.	May have some facial movements. Often, there are none, and the face appears still.	Irregular.	Infants react to sensory stimuli although responses are delayed. State change after stimulation frequently noted.	From the drowsy state, infants may return to sleep or awaken further. In order to awaken, caregivers can provide something for infants to see, hear, or suck, as this may arouse them to a quiet alert state, a more responsive state. Infants left alone without stimuli may return to a sleep state.

(Table 10 continued on next page)

Table 10. Infant State Chart (Sleep and Awake States) (continued)						
Awake States	Body Activity	Eye Movements	Facial Movements	Breathing Pattern	Level of Response	Implications for Caregiving
Quiet Alert	Minimal.	Brightening and widening of eyes.	Faces have bright, shining, sparkling looks.	Regular.	Infants attend most to environment, focusing attention on any stimuli that are present.	Infants in this state provide much pleasure and positive feedback for caregivers. Providing something for infants to see, hear or suck will often maintain a quiet alert state. In the first few hours after birth, most new-borns commonly experi-ence a period of intense alertness before going into a long sleeping period.
Active Alert	Much body activity. May have periods of fussiness.	Eyes open with less brightening.	Much facial movement. Faces not as bright as quiet alert state.	Irregular.	Increasingly sensitive to disturbing stimuli (hunger, fatigue, noise, excessive handling).	Caregivers may intervene at this stage to console and to bring infants to a lower state.
Crying	Increased motor activity, with color changes.	Eyes may be tightly closed or open.	Grimaces.	More irregular.	Extremely responsive to unpleasant external or internal stimuli.	Crying is the infant's communication signal. It is a response to unpleasant stimuli from the environment or from within infants (fatigue, hunger, discomfort). Crying tells us infants' limits have been reached. Sometimes infants can console themselves and return to lower states. At other times, they need help from caregivers.

Note. Adapted from *Neonatal Behavioral Assessment Scale* by T.B. Brazelton, 1984, 19. Philadelphia: J.B. Lippincott. © 1984 by J.B. Lippincott. Reprinted by permission.

Table 11. Newborn Screening Summary

Disorder	Basic Defect	Symptoms	+Screening Incidence	Criteria	Treatment	Follow-Up Needs
PKU (Classic)	Lack of enzyme to properly convert the amino acid phenylalanine to tyrosine.	Severe mental retardation, eczema, seizures, behavior disorders, decreased pigmentation, distinctive "mousy" odor.	1:10,000 to 1:15,000 More common in whites.	Elevated Phe.	Low phenylalanine diet; possible tyrosine supplementation.	Lifelong dietary management; careful monitoring of hyperphevariants; careful management and preconception counseling and intervention for PKU women in the reproductive years.
Congenital hypothyroid-ism (primary)	Absent or hypoplastic gland; dysfunctional gland	Mental and motor retardation, short stature, coarse, dry skin and hair, hoarse cry, constipation.	Overall 1:4,000 with ethnic variation 1:12,000 black 1:1,000 Indian.	Low T$_4$, Elevated TSH.	Replacement of L-thyroxine.	Maintain L-thyroxine levels in upper half of normal range; periodic bone age to monitor growth.
Galactosemia (transferase deficiency)	Absent or low activity of enzyme to convert galactose into glucose.	Neonatal death from severe dehydration, sepsis or liver pathology; mental retardation, jaundice, blindness, cataracts.	1:10,000 to 1:90,000.	Elevated galactose (Hill); low or absent fluorescence (Beutler).	Eliminate galactose and lactose from the diet; soy formulas in infancy; lactose-free solid foods.	Provide early monitoring for speech and neurological problems; educate parents about hidden sources of lactose; monitor females for secondary ovarian failure; avoid medications with lactose fillers.
Maple syrup urine disease (MSUD)	Absent or low activity of enzyme needed to metabolize leucine, isoleucine and valine.	Acidosis; hypertonicity and seizures, vomiting, drowsiness, apnea, coma; infant death or severe mental retardation and neurological impairment; behavioral disorders.	1:90,000 to 1:200,000.	Elevated leucine.	Diet low in leucine, isoleucine and valine. Thiamine supplement if responsive.	Educate family and friends regarding strict dietary regimen; social and education evaluation, behavioral counseling; neurological monitoring; prompt treatment of illness to minimize acidosis.

(Table 11 continued on next page)

Table 11. Newborn Screening Summary (continued)

Disorder	Basic Defect	Symptoms	+Screening Incidence	Criteria	Treatment	Follow-Up Needs
Homocystin-uria	Deficiency of enzyme cytothianine synthase needed for homocystine metabolism.	Mental retardation, seizures, behavioral disorders, early-onset thromboses, dislocated lenses, tall lanky body habitus.	1:200,000.	Elevated methionine.	Methionine-restricted diet; cystine supplement; B_6 supplement if responsive.	Maintain lifelong low methionine diet; monitor for thrombosis (check pulses, etc.) ophthalmological care; educational and psychological evaluation; avoid unnecessary surgery.
Congenital adrenal hyperplasia (CAH)	Defect in the enzyme 21-hydroxylase.	Hyponatremia, hypokalemia, hypoglycemia, dehydration and early death; ambiguous genitalia in females; progressive virilization in both sexes.	1:15,000 to 1:3,000 native Eskimos.	Elevated 17-hydroxypro-gesterone; abnormal electrolytes.	Replace corticosteroids; plastic surgery to correct ambiguous genitalia.	Maintain adequate corticosteroids; elevate doses or give injectable doses in times of stress; periodic bone age to monitor adequate treatment; maintain pediatric endocrinology follow-up appointments.
Biotinidase deficiency	Low activity of the enzyme biotinidase; biotin deficiency.	Mental retardation, seizures, ataxia, skin rash, hearing loss, alopecia, optic nerve atrophy, coma and death.	1:60,000 to 1:100,000.	Deficient or absent activity of biotinidase on calori-metric assay.	10 mg biotin daily	Monitor compliance; periodic followup and evaluation.

Note. From "Newborn Screening: The Miracle and Challenge" by L. Wright, A. Brown, and A. Davidson-Mundt, *Journal of Pediatric Nursing,* 1992, 7(1), 28. Reprinted by permission.

Sample collection for screening is most accurately done between 48 and 72 hours after birth...

Metabolic Screening

Newborn metabolic screening programs first became technically feasible in 1962 when Dr. Robert Guthrie developed a simple, cost-effective method of screening using a small amount of blood collected on filter paper (Guthrie & Susi, 1963). Screening programs are now mandatory in most states and are used to identify infants at risk for phenylketonuria (PKU), congenital hypothyroidism (CH), other inborn errors of metabolism, and hemoglobinopathies. Table 11 provides a summary of newborn screening tests for inborn errors of metabolism. These conditions can cause mental retardation, permanent disability, or even death if not diagnosed and treated promptly (Wright, Brown, & Davidson-Mundt, 1992). There is state variation regarding the conditions screened, methods, and types of tests.

Sample collection for screening is most accurately done between 48 and 72 hours after birth, which permits time for the normal metabolic changes that occur during transition to extra-uterine life. This time frame allows for the newborn to have ingested formula or breastmilk (protein) in order for the PKU screening test to be accurate, but is early enough to identify conditions such as Galactosemia and Maple Syrup Urine Disease before the onset of life-threatening symptoms (Wright, et al., 1992). When discharge occurs prior to 48 hours, an initial sample should be obtained. If the infant has not adequately fed, is being treated with antibiotics or is less than 24 hours old when tested, a second sample is needed. At least some states require that an initial sample be obtained immediately prior to discharge, with a second sample obtained at seven to 14 days of life (Wright, et al., 1992).

PKU has an incidence of 1:10,000 to 1:15,000 births (incidence higher among whites). PKU is a group of autosomal recessive disorders resulting in problems with phenylalanine metabolism. Early detection allows for appropriate dietary management, which prevents the irreversible complications of seizures and mental retardation. The prognosis is good for appropriate growth and development with relevant therapy; treatment consists of lifelong monitoring and dietary restriction of phenylalanine (Wright, et al., 1992).

Congenital hypothyroidism (CH) has an incidence of 1:4,000 with marked ethnic variation (Brown, Fernhoff, Milner, McEwen, & Elsas, 1981), and screening for this problem is combined with PKU testing in all states. CH is usually caused by an abnormally placed, hypoplastic or absent thyroid gland, but may also be the result of an abnormally functioning thyroid.

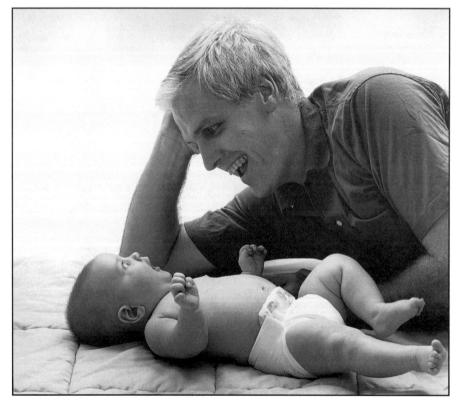

Untreated hypothyroidism results in mental retardation, short stature, and coarse, dry skin and hair. Infants who receive prompt intervention with supplementary L-thyroxine follow normal growth and development parameters.

The sickle cell diseases are hemoglobinopathies such as hemoglobin SS disease, hemoglobin SC disease and sickle-thalassemia. All result from the production of abnormal beta chains of hemoglobin. Thirty-six states have newborn screening programs for hemoglobinopathies (Wright, et al., 1992). The SS genotype causes sickle cell anemia, an autosomal recessive condition, and is the most common inherited disorder for which screening is available, with an estimated incidence as high as 1:400 in African-Americans. The sickle cell mutation is most common in persons of African descent; however, it is also documented in all groups from southern Europe, the Mediterranean basin, the Middle East, and Asia (Wright, et al., 1992). Symptoms of sickle cell anemia are due to either blockage of capillaries caused by misshaped red blood cells or from anemia secondary to red cell destruction. Symptoms range from mild, painful episodes to organ damage, stroke, shock and death. The SC form of sickle cell disease causes symptoms similar to sickle cell anemia.

The goal of early identification of newborns with sickle cell anemia is to prevent sickle cell crises. Family education regarding prevention strategies is appropriate. These include hydration to prevent stagnation of red cells and blockage of capillaries; acetaminophen for pain; penicillin prophylaxis beginning by two to four months of age; routine immunizations as well as pneumococcal vaccine; and avoidance of environmental causes of sickling, such as constricting clothing with elastic bands at the wrists and ankles,

and sudden temperature changes (Wright, et al., 1992).

The screening test for sickle cell disease is hemoglobin electrophoresis, which distinguishes fetal hemoglobin (F) and normal hemoglobin (A) from sickle hemoglobin (S). Newborn screening with hemoglobin electrophoresis identifies carriers as well as those with sickle cell anemia. The sample is either collected on the same filter paper used for metabolic screening or from cord blood at the time of delivery, depending upon state policy (Irons, 1993).

Neonatal nurses should be knowledgeable regarding the specific regulations that apply to their state screening programs, including for what disorders screening is offered; the signs, symptoms and outcome of untreated conditions; the criteria for repeat tests; available treatments; hereditary patterns; and the laws and policies of the state and institution regarding newborn screening (Wright, et al., 1992).

Perinatal Infections

Perinatal infections contribute to morbidity, mortality and increased length of hospital stay in newborn infants. The fetus and neonate are particularly susceptible to infection. Immune system development begins early in gestation; however, many immunologic responses are not functional or function inadequately by the early newborn period (Crockett, 1995; Blackburn & Loper, 1992; Lewis & Wilson, 1992). Incomplete mucosal defenses may allow the newborn to be more readily colonized by pathogens; even when infected, most newborns do not produce detectable type-specific antibodies; and newborns are unable to effectively localize infection because of the inability to produce adequate phagocytes and deliver

Neonatal nurses should be knowledgeable regarding the specific regulations that apply to their state screening programs...

them to the site of infection (Lewis & Wilson, 1992). The term newborn has some temporary passive immunity against infectious organisms to which the mother has antibodies, as a result of transplacental transfer of immuno-globulins, primarily IgG. Decreased levels of IgA result in reduced defense against gastrointestinal and respiratory infections, and decreased levels of IgM reduce the newborn's defense against viral and gram-nega-tive bacteria (Blackburn & Loper, 1992). Immunologic immaturity places the newborn at increased risk for the following:

- Generalized sepsis in the presence of bacterial infection
- Respiratory and gastrointestinal infections
- E. Coli sepsis, rubella, syphilis, toxoplasmosis, cytomegalovirus (CMV) and other viral infections
- Fungal infections

The newborn's increased susceptibility to infection and decreased ability to respond to it make risk assessment and early identification vital to reducing morbidity and mortality.

Predisposing general risk factors for infection in the term newborn may be maternal and/or neonatal (Askin, 1995; Witek-Janusek & Cusak, 1994; Lott, Nelson, Fahrner, & Kenner, 1993):

Maternal	Neonatal
• Maternal malnutrition	• Prematurity
• Lack of prenatal care	• Perinatal asphyxia
• Substance abuse	• Male sex
• TORCH infections	• Concurrent neonatal disease
• Peripartum maternal fever	• IUGR
• Clinical amnionitis	• Galactosemia
• Urinary tract infection at time of delivery	• Congenital asplenia
• Vaginal colonization with GBS	
• Perineal colonization with E. Coli	
• Prolonged rupture of membranes (> 24 hours)	
• Sexually transmitted disease	

Maternal infection can be passed to the fetus and newborn transplacentally in utero, at the time of delivery through direct contact with contaminated secretions in the birth canal, or after birth by contaminated breast milk (Remington & Klein, 1995). Intrapartal transmission of infection can occur through aspiration of infected amniotic fluid, or when vaginal flora ascend to the unprotected fetus following rupture of membranes during labor (Remington & Klein, 1995). Newborns with viral infections acquired during fetal life may exhibit no clinical disease, or they may demonstrate congenital malformation, intrauterine growth retardation, and chronic postnatal infection at birth (Remington & Klein, 1995; Strodtbeck, 1995).

Neonatal bacterial sepsis may be classified according to timing of clinical presentation. Early-onset infection usually presents within 24 hours of birth but can present up to the end of the first week, tends to progress rapidly, and has a 10%-25% risk of mortality even with appropriate therapy (Klein & Marcy, 1995). Bacteria associated with early-onset sepsis are usually those present in the maternal vaginal flora and include Group B streptococcus, H. Influenzae, Listeria monocytogenes, E. Coli and S. Pneumoniae. Late-onset sepsis usually presents after two weeks of age, but can occur anytime after the first week. It progresses more slowly and has a lower mortality than does early-onset infection, but a higher morbidity (Klein & Marcy, 1995). Organisms associated with late-onset infection include S. aureus, S. epidermidis, Pseudomonas and Group B streptococcus.

Assessment of risk for newborn infection begins with a review of the maternal history and intrapartum record for evidence of maternal infection. Maternal illness and infection during pregnancy should be documented on the prenatal record. Newborn assessment for clinical signs and laboratory analysis are important in diagnosis.

Group B Streptococcus

Group B Streptococcus is a gram-positive, anaerobic bacterium that colonizes the vagina or rectum of 10%-30% of pregnant women (Centers for Disease Control and Prevention [CDC], 1996). It is the most common cause of neonatal sepsis and meningitis in the United States. One to two percent of neonates born to women with GBS colonization develop early-onset, invasive GBS disease (CDC, 1996). Early-onset, invasive GBS disease accounts for approximately 80% of all neonatal GBS infections with a mortality rate of 5%-20% (American College of Obstetricians and Gynecologists [ACOG], 1996; Association of Women's Health, Obstetric, and Neonatal Nurses [AWHONN], 1996; CDC, 1996). Transmission to the fetus or newborn may occur during labor and delivery through direct contact with contaminated secretions or as a result of environmental exposure. Term newborns receive some passive immunity transplacentally when their mothers have type-specific IgG antibody to GBS strains (Blackburn & Loper, 1992).

Risk Factors. Major risk factors include preterm labor and birth, heavy maternal colonization, previous sibling with invasive GBS disease, prolonged rupture of membranes (PROM) >24 hours, and intrapartum maternal fever (AWHONN, 1996; Witek-Janusek & Cusak, 1994). Neonatal risk factors include prematurity, low birthweight and heavy surface colonization (AAP, 1997; ACOG, 1996; AWHONN, 1996; CDC, 1996).

Screening of pregnant women and use of prophylactic antibiotics have been controversial with separate recommendations from the AAP and ACOG. There

Assessment of risk for newborn infection begins with a review of the maternal history and intrapartum record for evidence of maternal infection.

Routine cultures of infants to determine GBS colonization are also not recommended (AAP, Red Book, 1997).

is now a consensus position presented by the CDC and approved by the AAP, ACOG, family practice physicians and nurse midwives (AWHONN, 1996; CDC, 1996, AAP, Red Book, 1997). The CDC issued recommendations for the prevention of early-onset GBS using one of two strategies, the first based on late prenatal culture and the other based solely on clinical risk factors. Intrapartum prophylaxis is recommended:

- When clinical risk factors are present, including a history of a previous infant with invasive GBS disease, GBS bacteriuria in the current pregnancy, delivery at <37 weeks gestation, duration of ruptured membranes >18 hours, or intrapartum temperature ≥100.4° F (≥38.0° C)

- When rectal and vaginal swabs for GBS culture at 35-37 weeks is positive

- If GBS status is unknown and membranes are ruptured ≥18 hours or IP temperature ≥ 100.4° F (≥38.0° C)

See Tables 12 and 13, Algorithms for prevention of early-onset of GBS using prenatal screening or clinical signs.

Management of newborns whose mothers receive antibiotic prophylaxis is based on clinical findings and gestational age of the infants, and routine use of prophylactic antibiotics is not recommended (CDC, 1996; AAP, Red Book, 1997). Routine cultures of infants to determine GBS colonization are also not recommended (AAP, Red Book, 1997). See Table 14, Algorithm for management of a neonate born to a mother who received prophylactic antibiotics in labor.

Newborn clinical signs may present rapidly within the first 12 to 24 hours

of life (often earlier for preterm and later for term infants) and include tachypnea, apnea, tachycardia, lethargy, pallor, cyanosis, temperature instability, poor feeding, irritability, seizures and jaundice (Askin, 1995; Witek-Janusek & Cusack, 1994). Early clinical signs may be subtle and nonspecific, making the maternal perinatal history important information in anticipating risk.

A complete blood count (CBC) with differential of the white blood cell (WBC) components is the initial laboratory screening tool when sepsis is suspected (Polinski, 1996). CBC findings suggestive of infection are listed in Table 15.

Neonatal nurses are often responsible for collecting blood samples. Since collection and handling methods can affect the quality of the results, knowledge regarding these effects is important (Hanson, 1994). Heelstick samples collected from unwarmed heels may give falsely high hematocrit or hemoglobin results because of hemoconcentration (Polinski, 1996). White cell counts have been found higher from unwarmed heel samples compared to venous and arterial samples and from specimens collected immediately after procedures that cause crying (Christensen & Rothstein, 1979). White blood count, neutrophil, and band counts were found in one study to be higher in term newborns born vaginally than in those born by cesarean (Hasan, Inoue, & Banerjee, 1993).

Implications for neonatal nurses include consideration of mode of delivery in interpretation of WBC and differentials, consistency of sampling site and technique to assess trends (Polinski, 1996), and allowing infants to rest one hour after procedures that cause crying (Christensen & Rothstein, 1979).

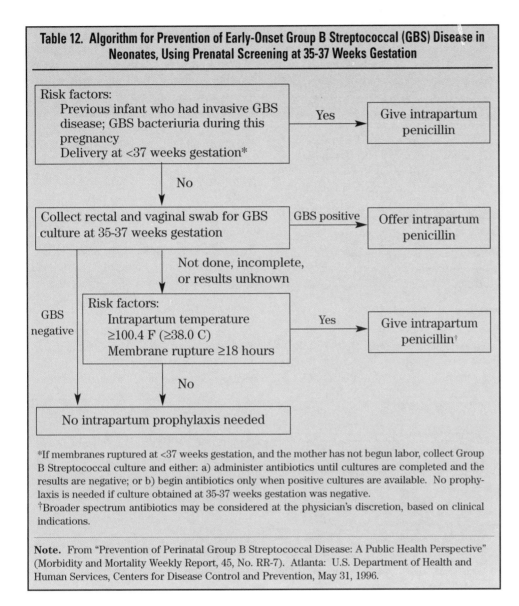

Table 12. Algorithm for Prevention of Early-Onset Group B Streptococcal (GBS) Disease in Neonates, Using Prenatal Screening at 35-37 Weeks Gestation

Risk factors:
   Previous infant who had invasive GBS disease; GBS bacteriuria during this pregnancy
   Delivery at <37 weeks gestation*

Yes → Give intrapartum penicillin

No

Collect rectal and vaginal swab for GBS culture at 35-37 weeks gestation

GBS positive → Offer intrapartum penicillin

Not done, incomplete, or results unknown

Risk factors:
   Intrapartum temperature ≥100.4 F (≥38.0 C)
   Membrane rupture ≥18 hours

Yes → Give intrapartum penicillin†

GBS negative

No

No intrapartum prophylaxis needed

*If membranes ruptured at <37 weeks gestation, and the mother has not begun labor, collect Group B Streptococcal culture and either: a) administer antibiotics until cultures are completed and the results are negative; or b) begin antibiotics only when positive cultures are available. No prophylaxis is needed if culture obtained at 35-37 weeks gestation was negative.
†Broader spectrum antibiotics may be considered at the physician's discretion, based on clinical indications.

Note. From "Prevention of Perinatal Group B Streptococcal Disease: A Public Health Perspective" (Morbidity and Mortality Weekly Report, 45, No. RR-7). Atlanta: U.S. Department of Health and Human Services, Centers for Disease Control and Prevention, May 31, 1996.

If mother and newborn are cared for by separate nursing teams, communication regarding mother and infant is imperative.

Nursing Management. Essential elements of nursing care include recognition of newborns at risk, and initial and ongoing assessments to facilitate early identification of infection. If mother and newborn are cared for by separate nursing teams, communication regarding mother and infant is imperative. In newborns receiving supplemental heat via incubator or radiant warmer, thermal instability may only be determined through careful monitoring of heater output. Penicillin or

ampicillin, along with an aminoglycoside, is the initial treatment of choice for a newborn with presumed primary sepsis. When GBS is identified as the causative agent, penicillin G or ampicillin alone can be given (AAP, Red Book, 1997; Cavaliere, 1995). The newborn may require no special diagnostic evaluation or treatment when the GBS-positive mother has received intrapartum antibiotic prophylaxis and labor and birth have been uneventful (Mahlmeister, 1996). Aside from routine universal precautions, no special precautions are recommended regarding isolation for GBS except in the case of a nursery outbreak of GBS disease (AAP, Red Book, 1997).

The ability of intrapartum chemoprophylaxis to protect the newborn from late-onset disease has not been established, so that discharge teaching must include written information regarding early signs of infant illness (Schuchat & Wenger, 1994). The neonatal nurse can simultaneously confirm that the infant has a primary pediatric provider whom the family can access after discharge.

Escherichia Coli

Escherichia Coli (E. Coli) is a gram-negative rod that makes up the majority of normal human fecal flora. It is the second most common cause of neonatal sepsis and meningitis in the United States (Askin, 1995; Guerina,

1991). Transmission is usually from mother to infant during labor and birth when the infant comes in contact with contaminated birth canal secretions. Sepsis or meningitis caused by E. Coli cannot be clinically differentiated from systemic infections caused by Group B Streptococcus and other infectious agents (AAP, Red Book, 1997).

Predisposing factors for neonatal Gram-negative infection include maternal perinatal infection, low birthweight, prolonged rupture of membranes, fetal hypoxia and acidosis, traumatic delivery, galactosemia, skin integrity defects (e.g., meningomyelocele) or asplenia (AAP, Red Book, 1997).

Nursing Management. Essentials of assessment and management for E. Coli sepsis are similar to Group B Streptococcal sepsis. Antibiotic treatment of choice begins with a combination of penicillin (usually ampicillin)

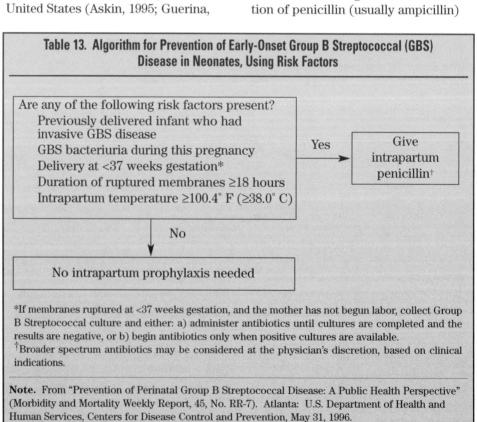

Table 13. Algorithm for Prevention of Early-Onset Group B Streptococcal (GBS) Disease in Neonates, Using Risk Factors

Are any of the following risk factors present?
  Previously delivered infant who had invasive GBS disease
  GBS bacteriuria during this pregnancy
  Delivery at <37 weeks gestation*
  Duration of ruptured membranes ≥18 hours
  Intrapartum temperature ≥100.4° F (≥38.0° C)

Yes → Give intrapartum penicillin†

No ↓

No intrapartum prophylaxis needed

*If membranes ruptured at <37 weeks gestation, and the mother has not begun labor, collect Group B Streptococcal culture and either: a) administer antibiotics until cultures are completed and the results are negative, or b) begin antibiotics only when positive cultures are available.
†Broader spectrum antibiotics may be considered at the physician's discretion, based on clinical indications.

Note. From "Prevention of Perinatal Group B Streptococcal Disease: A Public Health Perspective" (Morbidity and Mortality Weekly Report, 45, No. RR-7). Atlanta: U.S. Department of Health and Human Services, Centers for Disease Control and Prevention, May 31, 1996.

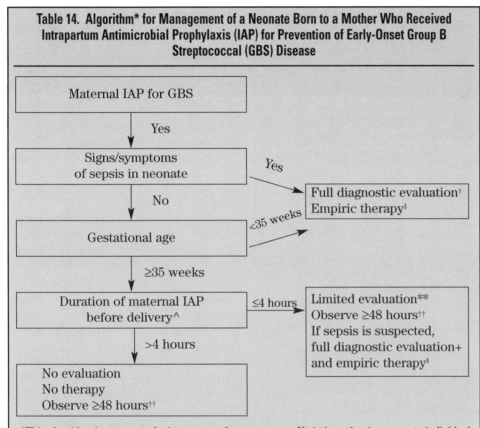

Table 14. Algorithm* for Management of a Neonate Born to a Mother Who Received Intrapartum Antimicrobial Prophylaxis (IAP) for Prevention of Early-Onset Group B Streptococcal (GBS) Disease

*This algorithm is not an exclusive course of management. Variations that incorporate individual circumstances or institutional preferences may be appropriate.

†Includes a complete blood count (CBC) and differential, blood culture, and chest radiograph if neonate has respiratory symptoms. Lumbar puncture is performed at the discretion of the physician.

§Duration of therapy will vary depending on blood culture and cerebrospinal fluid (CSF) results and the clinical course of the infant. If laboratory results and clinical course are unremarkable, duration of therapy may be as short as 48-72 hours.

^Duration of penicillin or ampicillin chemoprophylaxis.

**CBC and differential and a blood culture.

††Does not allow early discharge.

Note. From "Prevention of Perinatal Group B Streptococcal Disease: A Public Health Perspective" (Morbidity and Mortality Weekly Report, 45, No. RR-7). Atlanta: U.S. Department of Health and Human Services, Centers for Disease Control and Prevention, May 31, 1996.

and an aminoglycoside. Once E. Coli sepsis is confirmed, an appropriate cephalosporin (such as cefotaxime) may be used and/or an aminoglycoside, or both, if meningitis is suspected (Cavaliere, 1996; AAP, Red Book, 1997). Isolation or special precautions are not usually required beyond routine universal precautions.

Syphilis

Syphilis is caused by the spirochete Treponema pallidum. There are two modes of transmission: transplacental, or via direct contact with active genital lesions during vaginal delivery. At any stage of the disease, syphilis can be transmitted to the fetus. Untreated secondary stage in the mother presents the greatest risk for transmission

Table 15. Complete Blood Count Findings Suggestive of Infection

Neutrophilia (>13,000 WBC)

Neutropenia (<1,350 WBC)

Increased immature neutrophils (bands, metas, myelocytes)

Increased B:S (band to seg) ratio (>0.3)
Calculation = Bands divided by neutrophils

Increased I:T (immature to total neutrophil)
Calculation = % immature cells divided by (% Low or decreasing platelet count segs + % immature cells)1

Decreasing hematocrit

Note. Adapted from *Neonatal Infection: Assessment, Diagnosis, and Management* by J. W. Lott, 1993, 33. © 1993 by NICU Ink. Reprinted by permission.

(almost 100%) and causes the greatest risk of damage to the fetus, especially if it occurs during the period of organogenesis (AAP, Red Book, 1997; Lott, et al., 1993). Syphilis during pregnancy can cause preterm labor, PROM, stillbirth, congenital infection and neonatal death. Neonates born to mothers with late untreated syphilis usually present with no clinical signs (Lott, et al., 1993). When the infection is acquired transplacentally, newborns usually have signs of secondary syphilis with involvement of major organ systems.

Newborns with the following risk factors should be evaluated for congenital syphilis:

- Mother with untreated syphilis

- Maternal treatment not well documented

- Evidence of maternal reinfection

- Nonpenicillin drugs were used for treatment

- Mother is HIV seropositive

- Treatment is given within one month prior to delivery

- Maternal titers are unknown, stayed the same, or did not decrease with treatment.

Evaluation for congenital syphilis includes physical examination and serologic testing. Two types of serologic tests are used, nontreponemal tests and treponemal tests (AAP, Red Book, 1997). The nontreponemal tests commonly used to screen newborns for congenital syphilis are the VDRL slide test and the rapid plasma reagin (RPR) test. These tests measure quantitative antibody levels, which are helpful indicators of disease activity and useful to assess the adequacy of therapy. Neonatal serum is preferred to cord blood for testing, as cord blood can produce false-positive and false-negative results because of transplacental transfer of maternal IgG antibody (AAP, Red Book, 1997). Treponemal tests include fluorescent treponemal antibody absorption (FTA-ABS) test and the microhemagglutination test for T. pallidum (MHA-TP) and are used to establish a provisional diagnosis. Positive FTA-ABS and MHA-TP tests usually remain reactive for life. In a newborn with clinical findings suggestive of congenital syphilis, a positive VDRL and/or FTA-ABS test on serum provides strong evidence of congenital syphilis regardless of treatment received by the mother during pregnancy (AAP, Red Book, 1997).

Cerebrospinal fluid VDRL should also be examined in all infants born to mothers with syphilis during pregnancy and in those with suspected or proven congenital syphilis (AAP, Red Book, 1997). Results of CSF VDRL, however, can be positive in an uninfected newborn with a transplacentally acquired, high-serum VDRL titer. Long bone X-rays are not indicated if diagnosis is established by other studies. Determination of antitreponemal immunoglobulin M (IgM) antibody may also be included in the evaluation, if available.

Clinical signs are diffuse and include hepatosplenomegaly, jaundice, lymphadenopathy, IUGR, anemia, osteochondritis and vesicular bullous eruptions, which are most commonly seen on the palms of the hands and the soles of the feet (Lott, et al., 1993). Rhinitis or snuffles is a common early sign.

The drug of choice for treatment of syphilis at any stage is parenteral penicillin G. Recommendations and duration of treatment for newborns vary depending on clinical status and serologic indicators (AAP Red Book, 1997).

Nursing Management. In addition to universal precautions, drainage/secretion precautions are indicated for newborns with suspected or proven congenital syphilis until antibiotic therapy has been administered for a minimum of 24 hours. Gloves should be worn by parents, visitors and health care providers. Breastfeeding is not contraindicated for infants whose mothers have been treated (Crane, 1992; Starling, 1994; Tilman, 1992). Maternal education regarding effective treatment and long-term outcome is appropriate. Postdischarge followup is imperative for infected mothers and infants to ensure adequate treatment. Local public health authorities should be notified for tracking and followup. Confirmation of primary care providers for both mother and infant is also necessary before discharge along with communication regarding the need for serologic and other follow-up tests.

Gonorrhea

The causative organism species for gonococcal infection in the neonate is Neisseria gonorrhoeae, a Gram-negative diplococci. Intrapartum contamination of the newborn usually occurs during contact with maternal secretions in the birth canal, but can also occur in utero after rupture of the membranes. The most common clinical manifestation in neonates is ophthalmia neonatorum or conjunctivitis. Infection may also present as scalp abscesses (related to intrapartal scalp monitoring), vaginitis or systemic disease with bacteremia, arthritis, meningitis and/or endocarditis (AAP, Red Book, 1997).

Prevention of neonatal infection is the goal of management. Perinatal prevention strategies include routine screening of all pregnant women for gonorrhea at the first prenatal visit and second culture late in the third trimester for women at high risk of exposure; and neonatal prophylactic instillation of 0.5% erythromycin, 1% tetracycline, or 1% silver nitrate eye drops immediately after birth (AAP, Red Book, 1997).

Newborns at risk for gonococcal infection are those whose mothers have active gonococcal infection at the time of birth, a history in the current pregnancy of gonococcal disease with unknown follow-up status, received no prenatal care, have multiple sexual partners or are adolescent.

Nursing Management. Correct administration of eye prophylaxis will prevent gonococcal infection in most infants. Infants should be examined for clinical evidence of ophthalmia neonatorum (conjunctivitis), purulent discharge and corneal ulcerations, scalp abscess and signs of disseminated infection/ sepsis. If clinically indicated, cultures of eye discharge, blood and CSF are obtained to confirm

71

the diagnosis and determine antibiotic sensitivity. Ceftriaxone in a single dose (25-50 mg/Kg intravenously or intramuscularly for term newborns) is the recommended antimicrobial therapy for nondisseminated infections, including ophthalmia neonatorum, and for infants born to mothers with active gonorrhea at the time of delivery (AAP, Red Book, 1997). Cefotaxime in a single dose (100 mg/Kg) IV or IM is an alternative for ophthalmia neonatorum and is recommended for infants with hyperbilirubinemia. The eyes of infants with conjunctivitis should be irrigated with saline at birth and regularly until the discharge is cleared. Ophthalmic antibiotic ointment alone is not adequate for treatment, and is not necessary when appropriate systemic antibiotic treatment is given. For disseminated infections, ceftriaxone (25-50 mg/Kg IV or IM, once daily) for seven days, or cefotaxime (50-100 mg/Kg/d given IV or IM in two divided doses) for seven days is recommended therapy (AAP, Red Book, 1997).

Newborn infants with gonococcal infection, including ophthalmia neonatorum, should be managed with standard universal precautions (AAP, Red Book, 1997). There are no contraindications to breastfeeding with maternal gonococcal infection (Ingram, 1994; Judson & Ehret, 1994). Gonococcal infection must be reported to public health officials. In addition, communication with the primary pediatric provider facilitates followup for well-child care and ophthalmology.

Hepatitis B

Although five different types of hepatitis virus have been identified (A, B, C, D and E), type B (HBV) is seen most often in perinatal and neonatal infection. Hepatitis C virus (HCV) is also seen in the perinatal population, but transmission is relatively rare except in women with high viral titers and those with the

human immunodeficiency virus (HIV) (Alter, 1995; Freitag-Koontz, 1996).

The rate of perinatal HBV transmission is high (76%) in mothers with acute HBV in the third trimester or near the time of delivery, and low (10%) when HBV occurs in the first two trimesters (Zeldis & Crumpacher, 1995). Neonatal infection usually occurs at birth when the infant comes in direct contact with contaminated maternal blood and vaginal fluid. Mothers positive for hepatitis B surface antigen (HBsAg) are infectious, and those also positive for the envelope antigen (HBeAg) are highly infectious (Freitag-Koontz, 1996). Ninety percent of infants born to women both HBsAg-positive and HBeAg-positive are at risk for developing HBV during the first year of life if not treated (Lott, et al., 1993). The majority of infants born to women with HBV are asymptomatic at birth.

Prevention is the most appropriate course of action. Since 1988, CDC guidelines, including recommendations from the American Academy of Pediatrics (AAP) and the Immunization Practices Advisory Committee (ACIP), recommend screening for all pregnant women for HBsAg (CDC, 1988). Current guidelines recommend repeat HBsAg testing late in pregnancy for women who are HBsAg-negative but are at high risk of HBV (IV drug users, those with other sexually transmitted diseases) or who have clinical evidence of hepatitis (CDC, 1991; AAP, Red Book, 1997).

Any infant born to a mother who tests HBsAg-positive should receive both hepatitis B immunoglobulin (HBIG) and the first dose of hepatitis B vaccine within the first 12 hours of life, by intramuscular injection into separate sites. Subsequent doses of vaccine are due at one to two months and six months of age (AAP, Red Book, 1997).

Infants born to mothers whose HBsAg status is unknown at delivery should receive hepatitis B vaccine within 12 hours of birth (in the dose recommended for infants born to HBsAg-positive mothers). If the mother is determined to be HBsAg-positive, the infant should be given HBIG (0.5 mL) as soon as possible, but within seven days after birth. Subsequent vaccinations should follow the recommendations for infants of HBsAg-positive mothers (AAP, Red Book, 1997). For all other infants, three scheduled doses of vaccine should be given: the first before the infant's discharge from the hospital; the second at one to two months of age; and the last dose at six to 18 months of age. Two licensed vaccines are available in the United States, Recombivax HB and Engerix-B. Engerix-B is additionally licensed for an alternative four-dose schedule at birth, one month, two months, and 12 to 18 months of age (Freitag-Koontz, 1996). Dosages for Recombivax HB and Engerix differ and are listed in Table 16. If a 2.5 microgram (mcg)

dose of Recombivax is incorrectly given to an infant born to an HBsAg-positive mother, the vaccine should be administered again as soon as possible at the correct dose (5.0 mcg). An additional 2.5 mcg can be given if less than 24 hours have elapsed since the incorrect dose was given; otherwise, the full 5.0 mcg dose should be given (Freitag-Koontz, 1996). Breastfeeding is not contraindicated as long as the infant receives HBIG and the vaccine according to recommendations (AAP, Red Book, 1997; Freitag-Koontz, 1996; Hallam & Kerlin, 1991; Lott & Kenner, 1994a).

Nursing Management. Perinatal and neonatal nurses must be knowledgeable regarding perinatal HBV infection. Maternal screening information should be documented on the prenatal record. Nurses should be familiar with guidelines for prevention and prophylaxis for newborns of women who are HBsAg-positive or who have unknown HBV status. Specific issues for infants of HBsAg-positive women include the

Table 16. Recommended Doses and Schedules of Currently Licensed HBV Vaccines

	Vaccine	
	Recombivax HB (Merck Sharpe & Dohme)	Engerix-B (Smith Kline Beecham)
Age	Formulation/dose	Formulation/dose
Infants of HBsAg-negative mothers	Pediatric (brown) 2.5 micrograms (0.5mL)	Pediatric (blue) 10 micrograms (0.5mL)
Infants of HBsAg-positive mothers	Adolescent/high-risk Infant (yellow) 5.0 micrograms (0.5mL) or Pediatric (brown) 5.0 micrograms (1.0mL)	Pediatric (blue) 10 micrograms (0.5 mL)

Note. Adapted from "Prevention of Hepatitis Band C Transmission During Pregnancy and the First Year of Life" by M.J. Freitag-Koontz, *Journal of Perinatal and Neonatal Nursing*, 1996, 10(2), 40-55. © 1996, Aspen Publishers, Inc.

Current research into pharmacological prevention in the neonate is promising, most notably the administration of Zidovudine (AZT)...

following: (AAP, Red Book, 1997; Freitag-Koontz, 1996; Strodtbeck, 1995).

- Bathe infants after delivery to remove maternal blood and reduce risk of transmission

- Maintain standard universal precautions

- Educate mothers regarding HBV and the importance of a complete series of immunizations for their infants

- Provide written documentation of the infant's perinatal HBV exposure, and status regarding HBIG and vaccine administration on an immunization card with discharge instructions. Notify the infant's primary pediatric provider regarding the mother's HBsAg-positive status

Include in breastfeeding teaching the need to reduce the chance of cracked nipples, which might result in additional exposure of the infant to maternal blood and serous fluids.

HIV/AIDS

Human immunodeficiency virus (HIV) is a retrovirus that causes HIV infection and acquired immunodeficiency syndrome (AIDS). AIDS represents the most advanced stage of HIV infection. HIV infection may be transmitted from mother to fetus in utero transplacentally, intrapartally through contact with maternal blood, and from breast milk. Perinatal transmission is difficult to diagnose by standard immunoassays (ELISA and Western Blot) because maternal IgG antibodies found in the fetus and newborn result in nearly all infants born to HIV-infected mothers testing positive for HIV antibody at birth, while 20%-30% are actually infected (Miles, Balden, Magpantay, Wei, Leiblein, Hofheinz, Toedter, Stiehm, Bryson, & The Southern

California Pediatric AIDS Consortium, 1993; Shannon, 1995). Maternal IgG antibodies can be detected in the infant up to 18 months after birth. Determining true HIV status in infants has improved with the development of the polymerase chain reaction (PCR), HIV-p24 antigen and HIV cultures (AAP, Red Book, 1997; Miles, et al., 1993). The PCR detects the virus and not the antibody and is therefore not affected by persistent maternal antibody levels. The sensitivity of HIV-p24 antigen and HIV cultures is greater than the PCR. Using these nonantibody-based tests, most infected infants can be diagnosed by three to six months of age; however, only approximately 30% to 50% of infected infants will be diagnosed at birth (AAP, Red Book, 1997).

Women of childbearing age who are at increased risk for HIV include:

- IV drug users
- Those with multiple sexual partners
- Women who live in geographic areas with high incidence rates of HIV and engage in high-risk behaviors
- African-American and Hispanic women (CDC, 1994)
- Those with other sexually transmitted diseases

Neonates born to HIV-positive women are most often asymptomatic at birth, usually developing signs and symptoms between four and six months of age (Strodtbeck, 1995), but with a wide range of viral incubation of six weeks to 10 years (CDC, 1994). Clinical manifestations of HIV and AIDS in infants and children include generalized lymphadenopathy, hepatosplenomegaly, failure to thrive, oral candidiasis, recurrent diarrhea, recurrent invasive bacterial infections and opportunistic infections (AAP, Red Book, 1997).

Nursing Management. Prevention of HIV infection is the ultimate goal. Current research into pharmacological prevention in the neonate is promising, most notably the administration of Zidovudine (AZT) to pregnant women during pregnancy, labor and delivery, and to the neonate in the weeks after birth. Studies have shown a decrease in maternal-fetal transmission with such treatment, but long-term studies have yet to be performed. Specific nursing considerations include: (Judson & Ehret, 1994; Lott & Kenner, 1994b; Gunderson & Gumm, 1992):

- Strict adherence to universal precautions

- Bathing the infant as soon as possible after birth to minimize exposure to maternal blood and body fluids

- Breastfeeding is contraindicated in developed countries due to transmission via breast milk

- Maternal and family education regarding HIV infection and treatment

- Confirmation of primary pediatric provider and referral to a center for HIV followup and treatment

- Linking of family to support services

Treatment is supportive and based on clinical manifestations of the disease.

Tuberculosis

Tuberculosis (TB) is caused by the organism mycobacterium tuberculosis. The incidence of TB in the United States has resurged since the late 1980s, in association with the HIV epidemic, resulting in an increase in TB in young urban adults (Rosenfeld, Hageman, & Yogev, 1993). The increase in HIV-infected women of childbearing age, coupled with an increase in the incidence of TB in nonwhite women,

creates the potential for more pregnant young women to be infected with TB and to transmit the infection to their infants (Rosenfeld, et al., 1993).

Congenital TB, while rare, is thought to be transmitted by three possible routes: transplacentally from an infected placenta through the umbilical vein, ingestion of infected amniotic fluid, or inhalation of infected amniotic fluid (Smith & Teele, 1995). Neonatal TB can be acquired through inhalation or ingestion of infected droplets, ingestion of infected breast milk, or contamination of traumatized skin or mucous membranes (Smith & Teele, 1995). Epidemiologically, differentiating between congenital and neonatal TB is important; however, congenital and early neonatal TB have nearly the same presentation, treatment and prognosis (Rosenfeld et al., 1993). The term perinatal TB will be used here.

The incidence of TB is highest in urban, low-income areas and is increased in the following groups and situations:

- Foreign-born persons

- Migrant workers

- First-generation immigrants from high-risk countries

- African-Americans, Hispanics, Asians, American Indians and Alaskan natives

- Homeless persons or those living in a shelter

- Recent close contact with an infected person

- IV drug use

- HIV

Affected newborns are often born prematurely. Clinical manifestations are nonspecific: respiratory distress, fever, poor feeding, failure to thrive, lethargy, irritability and hepatosplenomegaly. Onset of signs and symptoms usually occurs in the first two months, with an average of two to four weeks. The Mantoux skin (purified protein derivative - PPD) test will usually be positive once the infant develops antibodies to the bacilli. Bacilli may be found in gastric aspirate, even when the PPD is nonreactive (Rosenfeld, et al., 1993).

Pregnant women diagnosed with active TB during pregnancy are treated with a recommended nine-month regimen of INH and rifampin. Although INH crosses the placenta, there is no evidence that it causes any risk to the fetus. There is also no reported increased incidence of congenital defects in infants born to women who received rifampin during pregnancy (Rosenfeld, et al., 1993).

Infants born to mothers who have completed treatment for TB and have no evidence of disease are at minimal risk and require no antituberculous treatment (Rosenfeld, et al., 1993). If the mother is being treated for TB at the time of delivery, the newborn should be evaluated carefully. Management of the newborn whose mother (or other household contact) has tuberculosis is based on categorization of the maternal (or household contact) infection. Refer to guidelines in the AAP, Red Book, 1997).

Nursing Management. Emphasis of nursing management includes protecting an infant from contracting TB from a mother with active or inadequately treated infection. The following interventions are appropriate:

- Bathing of the newborn to remove potentially infectious amniotic fluid

- Maintenance of standard universal precautions

- Prophylactic treatment of the infant with isoniazid (INH) and rifampin according to current protocols (Lott & Kenner, 1994b)

- Maternal and family education regarding TB, how it is spread and treated, with emphasis on the importance of fully completing treatment

- Skin testing of household contacts and, if necessary, X-rays and physical exams

- Followup with a primary pediatric provider in coordination with public health intervention.

INH is secreted in breast milk but no adverse effects on breastfeeding infants have been reported (AAP, Red Book, 1997; Smith & Teele, 1995). Transfer of the drug to the infant may be decreased by having the mother nurse or pump just before taking her own daily dose of medication in the evening and substituting a bottle for the feeding given during the night.

Chlamydia

Chlamydia is currently the most widespread sexually transmitted disease in the United States (AAP, Red Book, 1997). Chlamydia trachomatis is the bacterial agent most commonly found in perinatal infection (CDC, 1993; Lott & Kenner, 1994a). Transmission occurs at birth when the infant comes in contact with contaminated vaginal fluids in the birth canal. Acquisition occurs in approximately 50% of infants born vaginally to infected mothers and occurs in some infants delivered by cesarean with intact membranes (AAP, Red Book, 1997). The risk of conjunctivitis in those infants who acquire Chlamydia trachomatis is 25% to 50% and the risk of pneumonia is 5% to 20%. Conjunctivitis develops four to 12 days after birth. Treatment involves systemic pharmacologic intervention with erythromycin (50 mg/Kg/day in four divided doses) for 14 days; topical treatment is not necessary. Breastfeeding is permitted unless antibiotics used to treat maternal infection are contraindicated (AAP, Red Book, 1997; Hammerschlag, 1994; Judson & Ehret, 1994; Lott & Kenner, 1994a).

Herpes Simplex

There are two types of herpes simplex viruses, HSV-1 and HSV-2. HSV-1, usually transmitted horizontally via contact with oral lesions, causes fever blisters or cold sores. HSV-2 is usually transmitted via sexual contact and involves the genitalia. HSV-2 is the most common cause of disease in the newborn; however, HSV-1 accounts for an increasing amount of genital herpes simplex virus infections and does cause HSV disease in the newborn (AAP, Red Book, 1997).

Transmission usually occurs intrapartally with ascending infection, sometimes through apparently intact membranes or through contact with an infected birth canal during vaginal delivery. The risk of contracting the disease is higher if the mother is experiencing a primary infection (30% to 50% incidence), as opposed to a recurrent outbreak (less than 5%) (AAP, Red Book, 1997; Brown, Benedetti, Ashley, Burchett, Selkey, Berry, Vontver, & Corey, 1991; Carmack & Prober, 1993; Judson & Ehret, 1994). Postnatal transmission from mother and father to newborn is documented, including transmission by breastfeeding in the presence of breast lesions (Whitley, 1995).

Risk factors for transmission of HSV infection from mother to fetus/newborn include ruptured membranes, intrauterine fetal monitoring and fetal scalp sampling (Lott, et al., 1993).

Knowledge regarding maternal HSV status is vital in minimizing transmission and identifying infants at risk.

There is an increased incidence of prematurity and low birthweight. Clinical signs may be present at birth, and can take as long as three weeks to manifest. Symptoms are nonspecific and similar to those of bacterial sepsis; therefore, a thorough history must be obtained when trying to decide on a course of action.

Treatment includes antiviral pharmacologic intervention with acyclovir to optimize outcome and decrease sequelae and supportive therapy (AAP, Red Book, 1997; Whitley, 1995). There is no cure — and once infected, the virus will remain in the host forever with the possibility of subsequent reactivations. Long-term prognosis is good for infants whose infection is localized to the skin, eyes or mouth, but poor for infants with systemic disease (Brown, et al., 1992; Carmack & Prober, 1993; Judson & Ehret, 1994).

Nursing Management. The focus of nursing responsibilities for a family with HSV includes:

*   Careful history-taking regarding maternal and family HSV status

*   Thorough examination and ongoing assessment of the newborn

*   Maternal and family education regarding HSV infection in terms of mode of transmission and prevention, including careful handwashing prior to handling the infant

*   Instructing a mother (or father) with an oral lesion to wear a mask and refrain from kissing the infant until lesions have crusted and dried

- Isolation of neonates with HSV infection, or with positive cultures in the absence of disease, maintaining contact isolation precautions

- Permitting breastfeeding as long as no lesions are present on the breasts.

(AAP, Red Book, 1997; Lott, et al., 1993).

TORCH Infections

TORCH infections are caused by a group of organisms that are able to cross the placenta and harm the fetus. The acronym stands for the following:

T toxoplasmosis

O other (hepatitis, discussed previously)

R rubella

C cytomegalovirus

H herpes simplex (discussed previously)

Toxoplasmosis. The causative agent of toxoplasmosis is a protozoan parasite called Toxoplasma gondii. Human infection occurs after eating undercooked meat containing the cysts of toxoplasma, or handling soil or cat litter infested with the oocytes of the organism. Perinatally, it is transmitted via placental colonization from the mother to the fetus, and will only occur if the mother acquires the primary infection while pregnant (Grant, 1996). The intrauterine transmission rate increases with increasing gestational age, from 10% in the first trimester to 90% in the third. Fetal and neonatal morbidity and mortality increase with earlier transmission. Maternal infection after 24 weeks gestation usually results in mild effects on the fetus and newborn (Grant, 1996). Seventy to ninety percent of infected infants are asymptomatic at birth, but will develop symptoms within the first two months of life. Clinical signs and symptoms in the newborn include:

the classic triad of chorioretinitis, hydrocephalus, and intracranial calcifications, seizures, hepatosplenomegaly, late-onset jaundice, rash and petechiae secondary to thrombocytopenia (Remington, McLeod, & Desmonts, 1995). It is recommended that both symptomatic and seropositive asymptomatic infants be treated. Nursing management is supportive. No additional isolation precautions are recommended (AAP, Red Book, 1997). Breastfeeding is not discouraged unless antibiotics used in treatment are contraindicated (Bakht & Gentry, 1992; Hall, 1992).

Rubella. Rubella, or German measles, is a viral infection that can be transmitted via nasopharyngeal secretions, or transplacentally from the mother to the fetus. Immunization has significantly reduced the incidence; however, approximately 10% of young adults are susceptible to rubella, which creates potential for congenital infection (AAP, Red Book, 1997). Congenital defects following maternal infection vary widely depending on the timing of exposure. Most defects are associated with infection during the first trimester; thus, rubella titers are drawn on all pregnant women. The most common clinical manifestations of congenital rubella are cataracts, heart disease (patent ductus arteriosus or septal defects), neurological problems, deafness and low birthweight. Systemic infection often presents with purple lesions, or "blueberry muffin" rash. Prevention via immunization is the best treatment; treatment for active infection is supportive. Contact isolation in addition to universal precautions is recommended for congenitally infected infants. Infants with congenital infection shed virus in nasopharyngeal secretions and urine for one year or longer and should be considered contagious unless cultures after three months of age are negative. Breastfeeding is permissible after the infectious stage has passed in the mother (AAP, Red Book, 1997).

Cytomegalovirus. Cytomegalovirus (CMV), a member of the herpes family, is the most frequent cause of congenital viral infections in humans. Perinatal transmission is vertical through the birth canal or transplacentally, and may also be passed through breast milk (AAP, Red Book, 1997). In utero transmission can occur whether the mother had a primary infection or reactivation during pregnancy. Horizontal transmission can occur with exposure to infectious secretions.

Ninety percent of newborns with congenital CMV infection are asymptomatic (Strodtbeck, 1995). Clinical manifestations in symptomatic neonates include petechiae, microcephaly, hepatosplenomegaly, jaundice, intrauterine growth retardation, chorioretinitis and intracranial calcifications (AAP, Red Book, 1997; Stagno, 1995; Strodtbeck, 1995). The majority of congenitally infected infants appear normal at birth, but will develop signs later in life; the most common of these signs are progressive sensorineural hearing loss, mental retardation and developmental delays. Infected infants shed virus in their saliva for two to four years and urine for up to six years or longer, with the highest quantities of virus excreted in the first six months (Stagno, 1995). CMV is neither preventable nor treatable. Cytomegalovirus may be shed in breast milk; however, neonatal disease usually does not result, presumably because of transferred maternal antibodies (AAP, Red Book, 1997). Infants at higher risk include preterm infants and infants born to CMV-seronegative mothers who become CMV-positive during pregnancy. Parent education regarding CMV infection, viral shed-

ding and outcome is appropriate. Developmental and audiologic followup are important considerations of discharge planning for these infants.

Vitamin K Deficiency

It is estimated that one in 200 to one in 400 newborns not treated prophylactically with vitamin K at birth will develop Hemorrhagic Disease of the Newborn (HDN) (Snapp, 1996; Blackburn & Lopez, 1992). Hemorrhage occurs as a result of hypoprothrombinemia due to deficiencies in vitamin K-dependent coagulation factors (Greer, 1995). According to Blackburn & Loper (1992), the deficiencies in the various vitamin K-dependent coagulation factors (II, VII, IX, X) may result from: 1) poor placental transport of vitamin K; 2) lack of intestinal colonization by bacteria known to synthesize vitamin K; 3) maternal use of anticoagulants, anticonvulsants and antibiotics; 4) exclusive breastfeeding; and 5) history of perinatal asphyxia. In one study by Tulchinsky, Patton, Randolph, Meyer, and Linden (1993), two-thirds of infants whose deaths were attributed to hemorrhagic disease lacked vitamin K prophylaxis. Currently, some states have no health care codes governing vitamin K prophylaxis, and parents can refuse to have vitamin K administered to their newborns (Snapp, 1996).

HDN has been classified as Early, Classic and Late. Early HDN, seen in the first 24 hours of life, is the most uncommon. It is usually associated with maternal drugs (warfarin, anticonvulsants, antituberculous chemotherapy) but can be idiopathic in origin (Blackburn & Loper, 1992; Kisker, 1992; Moslet & Hansen, 1992). This form is often life-threatening and intracranial hemorrhage may be fatal. Classic hemorrhagic disease of the newborn occurs primarily in breastfed infants who develop hypoprothrom-

The Committee on Fetus and Newborn of the American Academy of Pediatrics recommends that every neonate receive a single parenteral dose... of prophylactic vitamin K₁...

binemia secondary to vitamin K deficiency. In the classic form of the disease, hemorrhage occurs between two and 10 days of life, and intracranial hemorrhage is uncommon (Greer, 1995). Generalized ecchymosis or gastrointestinal bleeding are the hallmark signs (Greer, 1995). Bleeding also commonly occurs from the circumcision site, urinary tract, umbilical cord stump and the skin (Clark & James, 1995; Greer, 1995; Kisker, 1992). Classic HDN is treated with parenteral vitamin K and there are no permanent sequelae (Greer, 1995). Late HDN occurs almost exclusively in breastfeeding infants who have not received vitamin K prophylaxis or in infants who have gastrointestinal disorders associated with significant fat malabsorption (e.g., cystic fibrosis, biliary atresia). Presentation occurs after the first four weeks and up to seven months of age (Greer, 1995; Kisker, 1992).

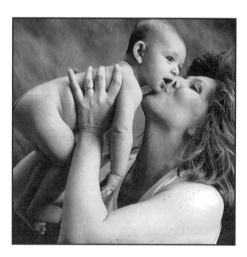

Laboratory diagnosis of vitamin K deficiency has traditionally relied on the indirect measurement of the various vitamin K-dependent coagulation proteins. Findings include prolonged prothrombin time (PT) and partial thromboplastin time (PTT) (Blackburn & Loper, 1992; Brown, 1992; Clark & James, 1995). Interpretation of these studies is complicated by the fact that

expected coagulation factors in the newborn are 30% to 60% of adult levels, so that prothrombin time is normally prolonged in the newborn as compared with the adult (Greer, 1995). One-stage prothrombin time is significantly increased only in instances of severe deficiency.

Prevention. The Committee on Fetus and Newborn of the American Academy of Pediatrics recommends that every neonate receive a single parenteral dose of 0.5-1mg of prophylactic vitamin K₁ oxide (phytonadione) at birth (AAP & ACOG, 1992). Controversy exists regarding vitamin K prophylaxis. In a recent study by Golding, Greenwood, Birmingham, and Mott (1992), the safety of the routine use of intramuscular vitamin K for the newborn was questioned because the researchers reported an increased rate of childhood cancer. Golding and colleagues (1992) concluded that the relative risk for some childhood cancers in the newborn who received intramuscular injections was significantly greater when compared to the oral or nonprophylaxis groups. Two subsequent population studies from Sweden and the United States refute the Golding study findings (Greer, 1995). The American Academy of Pediatrics Committee on Fetus and Newborn (1993) recently reviewed the status of prophylactic vitamin K administration in the United States and recommended that the present therapy with intramuscular vitamin K continue.

Recently, in cases where parents have declined the intramuscular route, the oral administration of parenteral vitamin K has been administered with no apparent side effects (Clark & James, 1995). Oral usage of parenteral vitamin K is not routinely recommended, however. Nursing considerations regarding administration of vitamin K are listed in Table 17.

Table 17. Nursing Considerations Regarding Administration of Vitamin K

1. Vitamin K is given as an intramuscular injection in the vastus lateralis muscle using a 25-gauge, 5/8 inch needle.

2. A one-time-only prophylactic dose of 0.5-1.0 mg is given in the delivery room or upon admission to the newborn nursery.

3. An additional dose may be given six to eight hours later, if the mother received anticoagulant therapy during pregnancy.

4. Observe for pain and edema that may occur at the injection site.

5. Observe for bleeding from the umbilical cord, circumcision site, nose, gastrointestinal tract, typically evident on the second or third day if it occurs.

6. Check that follow-up labs are ordered.

7. Give vitamin K prior to any invasive procedure (circumcision, spinal tap).

8. Vitamin K should always be protected from direct light.

Neonatal Polycythemia

Neonatal polycythemia is most commonly defined as a venous hematocrit of more than 65% (Werner, 1995). It occurs in 4% to 5% of the total population of newborns, in 2% to 4% of term, AGA newborns, and in 10% to 15% of SGA and LGA infants (Shaw, 1993). It has not been observed in newborns less than 34 weeks gestation (Shaw, 1993). Evidence of polycythemia usually presents within the first 48 to 72 hours of life.

The average hematocrit for term newborns on the first postnatal day of life is 61% (Oski, 1993) with a peak of up to 70% at two hours of age, followed by a progressive decrease through the first 24 hours (Werner, 1995). This initial rise in hematocrit is due to the movement of fluid out of the intravascular space.

Sampling site affects hematocrit values in the newborn. Capillary hematocrits (from heelsticks) are higher than venous values, especially during the early transition period when peripheral perfusion is sluggish. A venous hematocrit should therefore be analyzed when a high screening capillary hematocrit is detected.

Risk Factors. Risk factors for polycythemia include the following:

- Twin-to-twin transfusion, maternal-fetal transfusion and delayed cord clamping, resulting in increased fetal blood volume

- SGA, placental insufficiency and hypoxia, maternal diabetes, maternal smoking, maternal hypertension, maternal renal or heart disease, resulting in increased production of red blood cells (RBCs) in the fetus

- Placental infarction and previa, TORCH and other viral infections and postmaturity, resulting in uteroplacental insufficiency and increased production of RBCs in the fetus

• Genetic disorders such as trisomy 21, 13 and 18, and Beckwith-Weidemann syndrome.

Polycythemia may occur as a result of increased RBC production or secondary to red cell transfusion (Shaw, 1993).

Clinical Manifestations. Newborns with polycythemia are usually plethoric (ruddy) in appearance, and may be otherwise asymptomatic. Increased blood viscosity is the underlying mechanism responsible for clinically significant polycythemia. Hyperviscosity impairs peripheral blood flow, causing sluggish circulation. Eventually, the capillary circulation throughout the body is affected, compromising various organ systems (see Figure 17). Common central nervous system signs include lethargy, poor feeding, tremors and jitteriness; seizures and cerebrovascular accidents are rare (Werner, 1995). Hypoglycemia is the most common metabolic complication found in polycythemia; however, hypocalcemia is also seen (Werner, 1995). Hyperbilirubinemia associated with polycythemia results from destruction of excessive red blood cells. Cardiopulmonary findings include tachypnea, cyanosis and tachycardia. Pulmonary circulatory compromise can result in pulmonary hypertension, retained lung fluid and respiratory distress (Shaw, 1993). Hyperviscosity can also affect the kidneys, resulting in renal vein thrombosis and

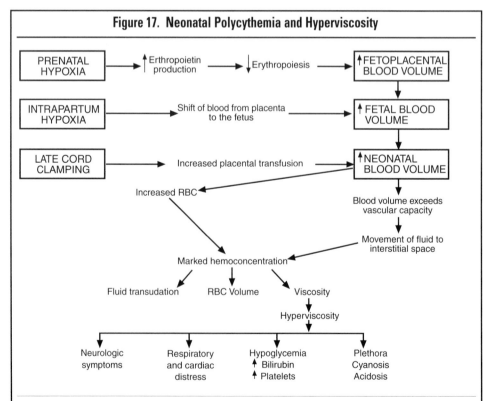

Figure 17. Neonatal Polycythemia and Hyperviscosity

Note. Adapted from "Neonatal Polycythemia and Hyperviscosity" by W. Oh, *Pediatric Clinics of North America*, (1982), 33, 523. © 1982 by W. B. Saunders Company. Reprinted with permission.

renal failure, and also the gastrointestinal tract, leading to necrotizing enterocolitis in term newborns.

The goal in management of polycythemia is to reduce the central venous hematocrit to less than 60% in symptomatic newborns. Treatment of asymptomatic newborns is controversial (Merenstein & Gardner, 1993).

Nursing Management. A screening hematocrit prior to six hours of age facilitates detection of a newborn with polycythemia and allows for appropriate management (Shaw, 1993). The newborn should be kept hydrated with monitoring of blood glucose and calcium levels.

Hyperbilirubinemia

Approximately 60% of full-term newborns become clinically jaundiced in the United States each year (AAP, 1994). Jaundice is characterized by yellow skin pigmentation resulting from increased levels of unconjugated bilirubin. Physiologic jaundice can result from expected changes in bilirubin metabolism that all infants experience. Some infants experience exaggerated physiologic jaundice from an excess of these expected transitional changes, while others experience additional problems that result in excess bilirubin accumulation and pathologic jaundice (Blackburn, 1995). Nurses who care for newborns should have a basic understanding of bilirubin metabolism and hyperbilirubinemia, knowledge regarding recognition of newborns at risk for developing hyperbilirubinemia and assessment skills for early detection of jaundice.

Several terms are used throughout the literature to discuss jaundice: physiologic jaundice, pathologic jaundice and hyperbilirubinemia. These terms are sometimes used interchangeably and with inconsistent definitions, making the understanding of jaundice more difficult (Blackburn, 1995).

Physiologic jaundice is an expected process that affects many term newborns. It usually presents during the first few days after birth, in association with a bilirubin level >5-7 mg/dl, as a result of normal physiological processes such as the metabolism of red blood cells (Blackburn, 1995; Maisels, 1994).

Pathologic jaundice refers to jaundice that occurs as a result of pathologic processes such as maternal-fetal blood group incompatibility, sepsis or excessive bruising that change the expected process involved in bilirubin metabolism (Blackburn, 1995).

Hyperbilirubinemia is defined as jaundice that occurs within the first 24 hours after birth, or persistent jaundice after one week in a term newborn, or excessive bilirubin levels (total bilirubin >12-13 mg/dl, direct bilirubin >1.5-2 mg/dl, or a rate of rise in bilirubin greater than 5mg/dl/day) (Blackburn, 1995; Maisels, 1994). This term is sometimes used to mean pathologic jaundice. It is more accurate to view hyperbilirubinemia as an increased bilirubin level that may be due to factors that can cause an exaggerated physiologic jaundice or pathologic jaundice (Blackburn, 1995).

Conjugated or direct bilirubin is bilirubin that has been metabolized or conjugated by the liver. It is water-soluble and passes from the liver via the common bile duct to the intestines for excretion. Most direct bilirubin is excreted in the stool. Some is reabsorbed in the colon and excreted in urine via the enterohepatic circulation (Blackburn, 1995).

Unconjugated or indirect bilirubin has not been metabolized by the liver. It is fat-soluble and not easily excreted in stool or urine. It poses the greatest risk for newborns because excessive accumulation results in deposition of unconjugated bilirubin in the skin, causing jaundice, and in the brain, where it can be toxic and lead to kernicterus (Blackburn, 1995).

Bilirubin Metabolism in the Fetus and Neonate. In utero, the majority of fetal bilirubin is unconjugated. It readily crosses the placenta and is excreted by the maternal liver. The newborn, therefore, is rarely born jaundiced.

Destruction of circulating RBCs accounts for approximately 75% of the bilirubin produced in the healthy

---

Figure 18. The Four Stages of Bilirubin Metabolism

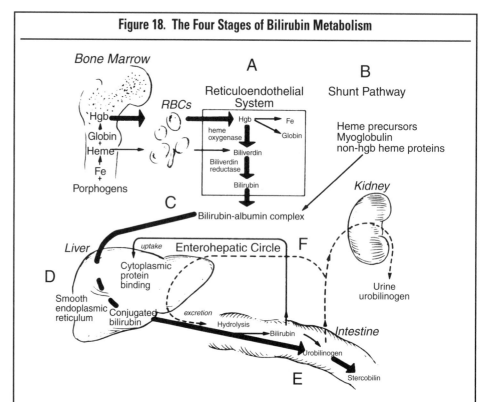

Production: (A) Hemoglobin is broken down into heme, iron and globin. Heme is further broken down by enzymes into biliverdin and then bilirubin (indirect). (B) Heme from nonhemoglobin sources is also converted into bilirubin. Transport: (C) Most bilirubin is carried in the blood to the liver bound to albumin; the rest is unbound or free. Conjugation: (D) The liver converts indirect bilirubin into water-soluble direct bilirubin, which it excretes into the intestine via the biliary tree. Excretion: (E) Direct bilirubin is converted in the intestines into urobilinogen and stercobilin. A small amount of urobilinogen may also be excreted in urine or returned to the bloodstream (- - - line). (F) Some urobilinogen is unconjugated by enzymes and converted back to indirect bilirubin. This indirect bilirubin is absorbed across the intestinal wall, reenters the circulation and returns to the liver (—line).

Note. From "Disorders of Bilirubin Metabolism" by L. M. Gartner and M. Hollander, M. In N. S. Assali, (Ed.), *Pathophysiology of Gestation*, Vol. 3, 1972, 457. © 1972 by Academic Press. Reprinted by permission.

term newborn (Blackburn, 1992; Nash, 1996). The process of RBC destruction occurs in the reticuloendothelial system and is a normal process that destroys aging, immature or malformed cells (see Figure 18).

Hemoglobin in the RBC is broken down into heme, globin and iron. Bilirubin is produced from the albumin complex breakdown of heme-containing proteins; 34-35 mg of bilirubin per gram of hemoglobin (Blackburn, 1995; Cloherty, 1991). Enzymes convert the heme to biliverdin and then to indirect bilirubin (Blackburn, 1995). A normal newborn produces on average twice as much bilirubin (6-10 mg/kg/day) as an adult (3-4 mg/kg/day) because of a higher concentration of circulating red cells, a shorter RBC life span (70-90 days), and limited hepatic enzyme production (beta-glucuronidase) (Blackburn, 1995; Jones, 1990; Wong, 1997).

Indirect (unconjugated) bilirubin is transported to the liver bound to serum albumin (see Figure 18). In the liver, a proportion of the bilirubin, but not the albumin, is transferred across the cell membrane into the hepatocyte. Indirect bilirubin and glucuronic acid then combine in the presence of the enzyme glucuronyl transferase to form direct (conjugated) bilirubin glucuronide. This conjugated bilirubin passes through the common bile duct and into the intestine, where it is reduced by bacteria and excreted (Blackburn, 1995; Nash, 1996; Ruchala, Seibold, & Stremsterfer, 1996). Reduced hepatic enzyme activity and reduced albumin binding capacity predispose the newborn to decreased capacity for conjugation of bilirubin. Bilirubin not bound to albumin is called free bilirubin. The amount of free or unbound bilirubin can rise when all of the albumin binding sites are used up, increasing the risk of jaundice and kernicterus.

Bilirubin Toxicity. According to Newman and Maisels (1992), term newborns without hemolysis are not at risk for brain damage or hearing impairment until serum bilirubin levels are greater than 20 mg/dl. Factors influencing bilirubin toxicity to the brain cells of newborns are complex and incompletely understood; they include those that affect the serum albumin concentration and those that affect the binding of bilirubin to albumin, the penetration of bilirubin into the brain and the vulnerability of brain cells to the toxic effects of bilirubin (AAP, 1994). It is unknown at what level or under what circumstances significant risk of brain damage occurs or when the risk of damage exceeds the risk of treatment (AAP, 1994). Concentrations considered toxic may vary in different ethnic groups and geographic locations (AAP, 1994).

Physiologic Jaundice
Physiologic jaundice can occur as a result of increased bilirubin production from hemolysis of RBCs, decreased albumin binding capacity, and functional immaturity of the newborn liver. Neonatal physiologic jaundice is usually a transient, benign condition that appears in the first two to three days of life and resolves within seven to 10 days. Almost all newborns experience elevated bilirubin levels but only half show observable signs. Incidence of physiologic jaundice differs markedly according to race. Infants of Asian descent, American Indians and Eskimos have a mean bilirubin level twice as high as whites. Blacks have a lower incidence than whites. In physiologic jaundice, serum bilirubin levels rarely exceed 15 mg/dl value (Hicks & Altman, 1993).

Almost all newborns experience elevated bilirubin levels but only half show observable signs.

Pathologic Jaundice

Pathologic jaundice can result from conditions that increase hemoglobin destruction, increase reabsorption of bilirubin from the intestine, impair liver conjugation, or interfere with liver excretion of conjugated bilirubin (Blackburn, 1995). Conditions that can lead to increased hemoglobin destruction include maternal-fetal blood group incompatibility (Rh, ABO), increased hemoglobin load from cephalohematoma and polycythemia, neonatal sepsis and congenital RBC abnormalities.

Other conditions that increase the risk of pathologic jaundice include:

- Passage of the first stool at greater than 12 hours after birth, resulting in increased enterohepatic circulation

- Drugs (morphine, phenobarbital, and certain antibiotics) that compete with bilirubin for binding sites on albumin, raising the levels of free bilirubin

- Births at high altitude that can result in increased bilirubin production accompanied by delayed bilirubin clearance in response to decreased oxygen availability and increased RBC production (McFadden, 1991)

- Asphyxia, hypoxia, hypothermia, hypoglycemia, which impair liver conjugation

- Congenital conditions such as biliary atresia and cystic fibrosis that can cause hepatic obstruction

Jaundice in Breastfeeding Infants

Jaundice associated with breastfeeding is characterized by an elevation in unconjugated bilirubin in otherwise healthy neonates. Approximately 6.8% of breastfed newborns develop unexplained serum bilirubin levels greater than 15 mg/dl (Maisels, Gifford, Antle, & Leib, 1988). Two patterns of jaundice in breastfed infants are described (Gourley, 1992):

- Early-onset, also referred to as breastfeeding or breastfeeding-related jaundice

- Late-onset breast-milk jaundice

Early-onset breastfeeding jaundice is the most common, usually becoming apparent between two and four days of life, and may be related to increased enterohepatic shunting secondary to decreased fluid intake and frequency of feeding of breastfed infants before maternal milk supply is established (Blackburn, 1995). Breastfed newborns with early-onset jaundice have bilirubin levels that are higher at three to four days and are more likely to develop bilirubin levels in excess of 12 mg/dl than bottlefed newborns. Breastfed infants excrete less bilirubin in their stools than do formula-fed infants. Decreased early stooling (the longer direct bilirubin remains in the intestine, the greater the probability that B-glucuronidase will convert it back to indirect bilirubin) and a longer period to establish gut flora (needed for further breakdown and excretion of bilirubin in the intestine) are factors that can also contribute to higher bilirubin levels seen in breastfed infants (Blackburn, 1995).

In breastfed infants with late-onset jaundice, the level of bilirubin rises between the fourth and seventh day after birth, when physiologic jaundice is disappearing (Brown, 1992). It occurs in one in 100-200 breastfed infants and is thought to be related to components of breast milk that interfere with bilirubin conjugation or excretion (Blackburn, 1995; Gartner & Lee, 1992; Maisels, 1994). Although factors in milk that produce jaundice have not yet been defined, investigation has centered on the roles of two observed effects of breast milk on bilirubin metabolism: inhibition of bilirubin UDP-glucuronyl transferase and enhancement of bilirubin absorption from the intestine. These may act alone or in conjunction to produce late-onset breast-milk jaundice (Whitington & Gartner, 1993). Clinically, the infant with late-onset breast-milk jaundice appears yellow on days five to six of life, which gradually resolves by three months of age (Gartner & Lee, 1992).

According to Buzby (1991), multiple studies have demonstrated support for increasing the frequency of breastfeeding as a measure to help reduce the total bilirubin serum level. Research has demonstrated that frequent breast-feeding (approximately 10 feedings per 24-hour period) is associated with adequate milk volume and reduced serum bilirubin level (Brown, 1992). It has also been proposed that early initiation and more frequent feedings may increase stooling and increase fecal bilirubin clearance (Brown, 1992). AAP guidelines for treatment of breast-milk jaundice are in Table 18.

Table 18. AAP Guidelines for Treatment Options for Breast-Milk Jaundice (1994)

- Observe.

- Continue breastfeeding; administer phototherapy.

- Supplement breastfeeding with formula with or without phototherapy.

- Interrupt breastfeeding; substitute formula.

- Interrupt breastfeeding; substitute formula; administer phototherapy.

Note. Treatment options for jaundiced breast-fed infants. (1994). *Pediatrics, 94(4)*, 561.

Early postpartum discharge complicates the management of jaundiced newborns because it places additional responsibilities on parents and guardians to recognize and respond to worsening jaundice or clinical signs. An indirect serum bilirubin level of 20 mg/dl is considered the upper limit, indicating immediate intervention if illness or associated conditions are present (Yeh, 1991). The infant should be assessed for a change in the CNS function, either depression or excitability.

Clinical Manifestations and Assessment of Jaundice. Jaundice in newborn infants can be detected by blanching the skin (AAP, 1994). As the total serum bilirubin level rises, jaundice develops in a cephalocaudal progression. There is also yellowish discoloration of the sclerae, nails and skin. Additional assessments should evaluate for bruising, activity level, feeding difficulties and behavior changes as well as other signs of problems such as sepsis, hypoxia, asphyxia, hypoglycemia and hypothermia, which are known to increase the risk of jaundice (Blackburn, 1995). Checking the maternal history for risk factors for jaundice allows for early risk identification and preparation.

Diagnostic Evaluation. The following recommendations were developed by the AAP to assist in the evaluation and treatment of the healthy term newborn with hyperbilirubinemia (AAP, 1994):

- Maternal/Perinatal testing: should include ABO and Rh(D) typing and serum screen for unusual isoimmune antibodies.

- A direct Coombs test, blood typing, and a Rh(D) type on cord blood should be done for mothers without prenatal care. The direct Coombs test is a measure of the amount of maternal antibody

Therapeutic management of the infant with hyperbilirubinemia is based on clinical judgment, history, course and clinical findings.

coating the infant's RBCs. When antibody is present, the test is positive. Infants with Rh incompatibility are direct Coombs positive; infants with ABO incompatibility have a negative or mildly positive direct Coombs test (Blackburn, 1995).

• Cord blood should be saved for the future, especially for those with mothers who have O-negative type blood.

• Assessment of the infant should be performed when family history suggests the possibility of glucose-6-phosphate dehydrogenase deficiency or some other hemolytic disease.

• A total serum bilirubin for infants jaundiced in the first 24 hours of life.

• A direct serum bilirubin level should be drawn if the newborn has a history of dark urine or light stool.

• If jaundice should persist longer than three weeks, a measurement of total and direct serum bilirubin should be obtained.

Therapeutic management of the infant with hyperbilirubinemia is based on clinical judgment, history, course and clinical findings. Potential benefits and risks of therapy should always be considered.

Phototherapy

Phototherapy is the application of fluorescent light on the infant's exposed skin. It is the most common treatment for hyperbilirubinemia. Mechanisms of bilirubin reduction by phototherapy are photoisomerization and photooxidation, which convert bilirubin to a soluble form for excretion. Guidelines for use of phototherapy are presented in Table 19. Intensive phototherapy

should be used if the total serum bilirubin (TSB) level does not decline under conventional phototherapy (AAP, 1994). If there is not a steady decline in TSB concentration, the presence of hemolytic disease or some other pathologic process is suspected and further investigation required.

Phototherapy is provided by bank bilirubin lights, spot lights and fiberoptic blankets. The effectiveness of phototherapy is not determined by the intensity of the light, but by the energy output from the light. Wavelengths in the 425-550 nm range are in the blue-green spectrum and are best absorbed by bilirubin. Equipment considerations are provided in Table 20.

Common side effects of phototherapy are generally transient and include thermal and other metabolic changes; changes in fluid status with increased insensible water loss; alteration in gastrointestinal function, activity and weight gain; potential ocular effects related to the lights and the use of eye coverings; skin, hormonal and hematological changes and psychobehavioral effects (see Table 21) (Blackburn, 1995).

Nursing Management of Infants Receiving Phototherapy. Nursing care of infants receiving phototherapy involves assessment of physical and neurobehavioral status; and interventions related to alterations in fluid volume, nutrition, skin integrity and thermal status (see Table 22). Emphasis is also placed on prevention of injury.

Fiberoptic Blanket. The Wallaby Phototherapy System is the most recent approach to the delivery of phototherapy in the hospital or home. Unlike the conventional phototherapy, the Wallaby System uses a fiberoptic blanket that comes in contact with the infant's skin, without danger of heat or

Table 19. Guidelines for Use of Phototherapy			
Term Infant <24 Hours	**Term Infant 24-48 Hours Old**	**Term Infant 49-72 Hours Old**	**Term Infant 72 Hours Old and Greater**
Jaundice before 24 hours of age requires further evaluation.	Phototherapy may be considered when the TSB level is ≥ 12 mg/dl, If TSB is ≥ 15 mg/dl, phototherapy should be implemented. If intensive phototherapy (multiple lights) fails to lower a TSB level of ≥ 20 mg/dl, exchange transfusion is recommended. If the infant is being seen for the first time and the TSB ≥ 25 mg/dl, intensive phototherapy is recommended. If intensive phototherapy is ineffective in lowering TSB, exchange transfusion is recommended.	Phototherapy may be considered in the infant with TSB level >15 mg/dl who is 49-72 hours old. Phototherapy is recommended when the TSB level reaches 18 mg/dl. If intensive phototherapy fails to lower the TSB level and the bilirubin level increases to 25 mg/dl, an exchange transfusion is recommended. If the infant is being seen for the first time and the bilirubin level ≥ 30 mg/dl, intensive phototherapy is recommended, and exchange transfusion should be planned for in case phototherapy fails to lower TSB level.	Phototherapy may be considered if the infant TSB level > 17 mg/dl. Phototherapy should be implemented if the TSB reaches ≥ 20 mg/dl. If intensive phototherapy fails to lower a TSB level ≥ 25 mg/dl, exchange transfusion is recommended. If the TSB level is ≥ 30 mg/dl when the infant is first seen, intensive phototherapy should be implemented while preparations for exchange transfusion are made. If intensive phototherapy fails to lower TSB level, exchange transfusion is recommended. Intensive phototherapy should produce a decline in the TSB level of 1 to 2 mg/dl within four to six hours and should continue to decline steadily. Bilirubin levels that persist above the level recommended for exchange transfusion after intensive phototherapy should be exchanged as per AAP guidelines.

Note. Adapted from Management of hyperbilirubinemia in the healthy term newborn by age (in hours). (1994). *Pediatrics, 94*(4), 560. Reprinted by permission.

Table 20. Equipment Considerations for Phototherapy	
Parameter	**Consideration**
Energy output	Irradiance of light source, not light intensity (illumination or brightness) determines effectiveness.
Irradiance levels	Effective range: 4-9 μW/cm^2/nm
Distance of light from infant	Amount of radiant energy delivered to infant is related to distance (increasing distance decreases irradiance; twofold increase in distance decreases irradiance fourfold); generally, lights should be 40-50 cm above infant.
Wavelength	Bilirubin absorbs light maximally at wavelengths of 425-475 nm (450-470 nm may be most effective).
Ultraviolet radiation	Reduced by placing a Plexiglass shield (1/4 inch thick) between light source and infant.
Electrical hazards	Units checked regularly for grounding and electrical leakage.
Effectiveness	Light emission may decrease over time. Monitor energy levels (irradiance) in the effective wavelength range and replace bulbs as recommended by the manufacturer.
Thermal hazards	Reduce risk of overheating or hyperthermia by monitoring of infant's thermal status and maintaining a space of about 2 inches between the incubator hood and lamp cover to allow free flow of air. Increased risk of overheating in radiant warmers with three-sided lights, which prevent radiant heat loss.
Alteration in blood values	Turn phototherapy off while blood for bilirubin samples is drawn.

Note. From *Maternal, Fetal, and Neonatal Physiology: A Clinical Perspective* by S. T. Blackburn and D. L. Loper, 1992, 650. © 1992 by W. B. Saunders. Reprinted by permission.

electricity, and does not require the use of eye shields when the blanket is snugly wrapped around the infant's torso (McFadden, 1991).

Nursing Management. The nurse should identify neonates at risk for developing kernicterus (history of acidosis, asphyxia, cold stress, prematurity, treatment with sulfonamides).

Assess the neonate for jaundice at least q4-8h, particularly the sclerae, skin over the forehead, and trunk. Ensure that appropriate serum bilirubin monitoring is done. If phototherapy is ordered, protect the newborn's eyes from phototherapy with eye shields, ensuring that the shield does not slip over the nose and obstruct the airway.

Table 21. Side Effects of Phototherapy		
Side Effect	**Specific Change**	**Implication**
Thermal and other metabolic changes	Increased environmental and body temperature Increased oxygen consumption Increased respiratory rate Increased skin blood flow	Influenced by maturity, caloric intake (energy to respond to thermal changes), adequacy of heat dissipation from phototherapy unit, distance of unit from infant and incubator hood (space for air flow, radiant heat loss), use of servocontrol
Fluid status	Increased peripheral blood flow Increased insensible water loss	Increased fluid loss May alter uptake of IM medications Due to increases in evaporative water loss, metabolic rate, and possible respiratory rate Influenced by environment (air flow, humidity, temperature); characteristics of phototherapy unit (heat dissipation, distance from infant); ambient temperature alteration; infant alterations in skin and core temperature, heart and respiratory rates, metabolic rate, caloric intake; type of bed (increased with radiant warmer and incubator)
Gastrointestinal function	Increased number, frequency of stools Watery, greenish-brown stools Decreased time for intestinal transit Decreased absorption; retention of nitrogen, water, electrolytes Altered lactose activity, riboflavin	May be related to increased bile flow, which stimulates GI activity Increases stool water loss Increases stool water loss and risk of dehydration Temporary lactose intolerance with decreased lactase at epithelial brush border and increased frequency and water content of stools
Altered activity	Lethargy or irritability Decreased eagerness to feed	May impact on parent-infant interaction May alter fluid and caloric intake
Altered weight gain	Decreased initially but generally catches up in two to four weeks	Due to poor feeding and increased GI losses
Ocular effects	Not documented in humans, but continued concerns about effects of light vs. effects of eye patches	Lack of appropriate sensory input and stimulation Eye patches increase risk of infection, corneal abrasion, increased intracranial pressure (if too tight)
Skin changes	Tanning Rashes Burns Bronze baby syndrome	Due to induction of melanin synthesis or dispersion by UV light Due to injury to skin mast cells with release of histamine; erythema from UV light From excessive exposure to shortwave emissions from flourescent light Due to decreased hepatic excretion of bilirubin photodegradation by-products (especially in infants with elevated direct bilirubin)
Hormonal changes	Alterations in serum gonadotropins (increased luteinizing and follicle-stimulating hormones)	Significance unclear May also affect circadian rhythms (unclear)
Hematological changes	Increased rate of platelet turnover Injury to circulating RBCs with decreased potassium and increased ATP* activity	May be a problem in infants with low platelets and sepsis May lead to hemolysis, increased energy needs
Psychobehavioral concerns	Isolation/lack of usual sensory experiences, including visual deprivation Alteration in state and neurobehavioral organization	Impact can be mediated by provision of appropriate nursing care May interfere with parent-infant interaction and increase parental stress

*ATP = adenosine triphosphate

Note. From *Maternal, Fetal, and Neonatal Physiology: A Clinical Perspective* by S. T. Blackburn and D. L. Loper, 1992, 649. ©1992 by W. B. Saunders. Reprinted by permission.

Table 22. Nursing Management of Infants Undergoing Phototherapy	
Nursing Assessment	
Area	**Parameter**
Physical status	Intake and output
	Color
	Location of jaundice
	Skin integrity
	Stools (character, consistency)
	Vital signs
	Infant/environment temperature
	Hydration status
	Signs of phototherapy side effects
	Eye discharge and tearing
	Position
	Activity
Neurobehavioral status	Sleep-wake states
	Sensory threshold
	Behavioral responsiveness
	Feeding behaviors
	Consoling abilities
	Stress responses
	Interactive capabilities
Nursing Management	
Nursing Diagnosis	**Intervention**
Fluid volume deficit (actual or potential)	Monitor intake and output
	Monitor hydration status (weight, specific gravity, urine output)
	Monitor stooling pattern, character
	Maintain adequate fluid intake (oral or parenteral)
Alteration in nutrition	Assess feeding behavior and activity
	Monitor fluid and caloric intake, weight, abdominal girth
	Remove eye shields during feeding
	Hold during oral feedings as health and thermal status permit
	Bring to alert state prior to feeding
	Feed on demand if possible
Impaired skin integrity	Observe color, rashes, excoriation
	Clean skin with warm water
	Clean perineal area after stooling
	Turn frequently (also increases skin exposure to phototherapy)
	Ensure plexiglas shield is in place between light source and infant to reduce exposure to UV light

(Table 22 continued on next page)

Table 22. Nursing Management of Infants Undergoing Phototherapy (continued)	
	Nursing Management
Nursing Diagnosis	**Intervention**
Potential for injury	Observe for side effects associated with phototherapy
	Observe for signs of sepsis
	Provide care to minimize side effects of phototherapy
	Shield eyes from lights with opaque patches
	Ensure eyelids are closed when shield is applied to prevent corneal injury
	Remove eye shield and observe eyes regularly
	Monitor position of eye shield to prevent occlusion of nose
	Avoid tight headband on eye shield to reduce risk of increased intracranial pressure, especially in preterm infants
	Observe for eye discharge, tearing
	Shield testes and possibly ovaries (data unclear about need to do this) with diaper
Alteration in thermal status	Place in warm, thermoneutral environment
	Monitor environmental and infant temperature
	Observe for hypo- and hyperthermia
	Reduce heat losses from environmental sources
	Use servocontrol for infants in incubator or under radiant warmer
	Shield servocontrol thermistor from direct exposure to phototherapy lights

Note. Adapted from S. Blackburn,. (1995). Hyperbilirubinemia and neonatal jaundice. *Neonatal Network, 14*(7), 15-25. Adapted by permission.

Assessment of parental understanding of the neonate's condition and therapeutic needs is imperative.

The eyes should be inspected for injury q4-8h with phototherapy lights off. Any form of discharge from the eye should be cleaned with sterile water. The newborn should be maintained at an appropriate distance from the lights, according to manufacturer's guidelines, and turned q2h. For quality assurance, documentation of the number of hours each lamp is used and changing the lamps according to the recommendation are necessary to maintain effectiveness. Since adequate hydration enhances bilirubin excretion, the newborn who is under phototherapy should be fed at least q4h. The hydration status of the newborn should be monitored by fluid and nutritional intake, urine and fecal loss, skin turgor, daily weights, serum electrolytes and urine-specific gravity. It is important that thermal stability be maintained and temperature monitored q2h and prn.

Assessment of parental understanding of the neonate's condition and therapeutic needs is imperative. Parents should be given the opportunity to be involved in the tasks of parenting such as feeding, bathing and providing comfort to the newborn. The nurse should encourage questions, and all information should be reinforced or clarified with parents. The nurse should discuss home management of mild to moderate physiologic jaundice, including frequency and volume of feedings, exposure to sunlight, and follow-up serum testing programs.

Summary

The term newborn is most often born healthy, making a complex but successful transition from fetus to newborn. Identifying risk in the newborn is enhanced by the availability of perinatal data, astute assessments during the immediate newborn period, and knowledge regarding expected norms and specific threats for newborns during the first days of life. Nursing assessments and interventions regarding transition to extrauterine life, hypoglycemia and thermoregulation are vital to the well-being of newborns and can significantly affect newborn outcomes. Additional assessments of newborn behavior and function provide important information about the newborn's transition period and ability to interact with the environment and caregivers. How an infant feeds, sleeps, awakens and responds indicates newborn stability and well-being.

Changes in those parameters may be early signs of alterations in health and are observations most appropriately made by knowledgeable nurses. Knowledge of the newborn period is essential for the perinatal nurse who may provide additional assessment data used to determine infant readiness and safety for discharge. Family education and anticipatory guidance can more readily be provided by nurses who understand and can articulate the rationale for metabolic screenings, vitamin K prophylaxis and infection prevention. Factual knowledge regarding jaundice in newborns can help facilitate timely and appropriate treatment as well as minimize the risk of complications. Knowledgeable perinatal nurses can contribute greatly to risk assessment and management during the immediate newborn period, minimizing the potential for complications and optimizing outcomes.

The following activities will aid the learner in applying some of the concepts presented in this module.

1. Review your unit's standard of care on thermal management of a patient receiving phototherapy in an isolette or warmer bed. Do these guidelines address thermoregulation? How?

2. What guidelines are available to monitor hyperbilirubinemia in the neonate discharged home?

3. What resources are available in your community for follow-up management of hyperbilirubinemia in patients who were discharged early from the hospital?

4. What is the standard of care for managing the neonate with hypoglycemia in your institution?

The following discussion points will aid the learner in applying some of the concepts presented in this module.

1. Describe what mechanism in your facility is in place to prevent heat loss in the delivery room for the term newborn.

2. How are infants with hypoglycemia handled in your institution? What are the guidelines for management of the patients with hypoglycemia and hyperglycemia?

3. How are patients with polycythemia managed in your facility?

Organizations

Association of Women's Health, Obstetric, and Neonatal Nurses
700 14th Street, NW., Suite 600
Washington, D.C. 20005-2006
(800) 673-8499 (US)
(800) 245-0231 (Canada)
Fax: (202) 737-0575
www.awhonn.org

March of Dimes
1275 Mamaroneck Avenue
White Plains, NY 10605
Phone: (888) 663-4637
Fax: (914) 997-4763
www.modimes.org
E-mail: resourcecenter@modimes.org

National Association of Neonatal Nurses
1304 Southpoint Boulevard, Suite 800
Petaluma, CA 94454
Phone: (707) 762-5588
Fax: (707) 762-0401
www.nann.org

Reading Material

Association of Women's Health, Obstetric, and Neonatal Nurses (AWHONN) and National Association of Neonatal Nursing Joint Task Force. (1997). *Neonatal nursing: Orientation and development for registered and advanced practice nurses in basic and intensive care settings.* Washington DC: Author.

Assessment of Risk in the Term Newborn

To receive continuing education credit for completion of this module via independent study, record answers to the following questions on the application provided and submit to March of Dimes for grading. Submission instructions are found on the application.

1. An infant classified preterm is born:
   A. Prior to the age of viability
   B. Between the 38th and 39th weeks of gestation
   C. Any time before the expected date of delivery
   D. Before completion of the 37th week of gestation

2. When assessing a newborn for physical maturity, an observation that supports prematurity is:
   A. Firm, large, protruding pinnae of the ears
   B. Fine hair over the middle of the back and shoulders
   C. Plantar creases that cover the anterior 2/3 of the feet
   D. Skin that is thick and flaky with veins that are difficult to see

3. Newborns who are small for gestational age are at increased risk for:
   A. Cephalhematoma
   B. Hyperglycemia
   C. Hypothermia
   D. Anemia

4. At birth, a newborn's assessment reveals a heart rate of 140, loud crying, some flexion of the arms and legs, withdrawal of the feet when stimulated, and a pink body with blue extremities. This newborn's Apgar score is:
   A. 5
   B. 6
   C. 7
   D. 8

5. Intrapartum antibiotic prophylaxis is recommended for Group B Streptococcus infection when the mother's:
   A. History reveals antibiotic prophylaxis in the first trimester
   B. Membranes have been ruptured for longer than 18 hours
   C. Length of pregnancy is greater than 40 weeks
   D. Intrapartal temperature is higher than 99° F

6. When assessing the pattern of sleep and activity in a term newborn, the infant is alert, heart and respiratory rates have stabilized, and meconium has been passed. The nurse determines that the newborn is in the:
   A. Second period of reactivity
   B. Initial period of reactivity
   C. Period of relative inactivity
   D. Transitional period of inactivity

7. Metabolic screening of newborns is primarily performed because:
   A. Early treatment can prevent disability
   B. Screening programs are mandatory in most states
   C. Diagnostic procedures are easy to perform in the hospital
   D. There is an increased incidence of metabolic problems in newborns

8. The manufacture of glucose from noncarbohydrate sources is known as:
   A. Fat mobilization
   B. Glycogen storage
   C. Gluconeogenesis
   D. Glycogenolysis

9. Transient neonatal hypoglycemia can be caused by:
   A. Hypoplasia
   B. Hypothermia
   C. Hypothyroidism
   D. Hypopituitarism

10. Newborns who are at risk for developing hyperglycemia should be assessed for signs of:
    A. Osmotic diuresis
    B. Ineffective feeding
    C. Respiratory distress
    D. Cardiac dysrhythmias

11. Which factor is specifically associated with pathologic jaundice?
    A. ABO incompatibility
    B. Functional immaturity of the liver
    C. Decreased albumin binding capacity
    D. Lowered hemoglobin load from polycythemia

12. When receiving phototherapy, the newborn should be monitored for side effects which include:
    A. Peripheral edema
    B. Eagerness to feed
    C. Decreased respirations
    D. Increased number of stools

13. A cool environmental temperature can cause heat loss in the newborn by the mechanism of:
    A. Radiation
    B. Convection
    C. Conduction
    D. Evaporation

14. To prevent heat loss in the newborn via conduction, the nurse should:
    A. Swaddle the newborn with a blanket
    B. Place the newborn on a warm surface
    C. Transport the newborn in an incubator
    D. Dry the newborn immediately after bathing

15. Newborns with polycythemia should be monitored for:
    A. Polyuria
    B. Bradycardia
    C. Hypocalcemia
    D. Hyperglycemia

Assessment of Risk in the Term Newborn

To receive continuing education credit for registered nurses and certified nurse-midsives via independent study of the *Assessment of Risk in the Term Newborn* **nursing module:**

1. Complete the registration information.
2. Legibly write the letter of the appropriate answer for each question in the space provided below.
3. Sign and date the application.
4. Return this application, the tear-out self-mailer evaluation, and a check for $35.00 made payable to **March of Dimes** to:
   Nursing Modules, March of Dimes, 1275 Mamaroneck Avenue, White Plains, NY 10605.

March of Dimes will notify you of your results within four to six weeks of receiving your completed test. If you receive a passing score (70%), you will receive a certificate of completion indicating the amount of continuing education earned. If your score is less than 70%, you will be given a second opportunity to pass the test.

This Educational Design II is provided by the March of Dimes Birth Defects Foundation, which has been approved as a provider of continuing education by the New York State Nurses Association's Council on Continuing Education, which is accredited by the American Nurses' Credentialing Center's Commission on Accreditation. **It has been assigned code MRCHDIMES-PRV-97-9736 and has been approved for 5.0 contact hours for registered nurses.** *It is also approved by the California Board of Registered Nursing, Provider #CEP-11444.*

REGISTRATION INFORMATION

Last Name _____ First Name _____

Social Security # _____ Credentials _____

Address _____

City _____ State _____ ZIP _____

Telephone _____ Fax _____

E-mail _____

INDEPENDENT STUDY TEST ANSWERS

1. _____	5. _____	9. _____	13. _____
2. _____	6. _____	10. _____	14. _____
3. _____	7. _____	11. _____	15. _____
4. _____	8. _____	12. _____	

Signature _____ Date _____

CHECKLIST FOR MAILING

☐ Completed (and signed) application

☐ Completed evaluation

☐ Check for $35 made payable to **March of Dimes**

Alexander, G.R., & Allen, M.C. (1996). Conceptualization, measurement, and use of gestational age. *Journal of Perinatology, 16*(1), 53-59.

Alexander, G.R., de Caunes, F., Hulsey, T.C., Tompkins, M.E., & Allen, M. (1992). Validity of postnatal assessments of gestational age: A comparison of the method of Ballard et al. and early ultrasonography. *American Journal of Obstetrics and Gynecology, 166*, 891-895.

Alford, C.A., Stagno, S., Pass, R.F., & Britt, W.J. (1990). Congenital and perinatal cytomegalovirus infections. *Review of Infectious Diseases, 12*(S7), S745-753.

Alter, H. (1995). To C or not to C: These are the questions. *Blood, 85,* 1681-1695.

Altimier, L.B., & Roberts, W. (1996). One touch II hospital system for correlation with serum glucose value. *Neonatal Network, 15*(2), 15-26.

American Academy of Pediatrics. (1994). Pediatric parameter: Management of hyperbilirubinemia in healthy term newborn. *Pediatrics, 94*(4).

American Academy of Pediatrics. (1997). Summaries of infectious diseases. In G. Peter (Ed.), *1994 Red Book: Report of the committee on infectious diseases* (24th ed.). Elk Grove Village, IL: Author.

American Academy of Pediatrics, American College of Obstetricians and Gynecologists. Relationship between perinatal factors and neurologic outcome. (1992). L. Poland & R.K. Freeman (Eds.), *Guidelines for perinatal care* (3rd ed.). Elk Grove Village, IL.

American Academy of Pediatrics Committee on Fetus and Newborn. (1995). Hospital stay for healthy term newborns. *Pediatrics, 96*(4), 788-790.

American Academy of Pediatrics Committee on Fetus and Newborn. (1993). Vitamin K ad hoc task force, AAP: Controversies concerning vitamin K and the newborn. *Pediatrics, 91,* 1001-1003.

American Academy of Pediatrics, Committee on Fetus and Newborn, & American College of Obstetricians and Gynecologists, Committee on Obstetric Practice. (1996). Use and abuse of the Apgar score. *Pediatrics, 98,* 141-142.

American College of Obstetricians and Gynecologists. (1996). *Committee Opinion: Prevention of early-onset group B streptococcal disease in newborns* (173). Washington, DC: Author.

Amspacher, K.A. (1992). Meeting the challenge of neonatal hypoglycemia. *Journal of Perinatal and Neonatal Nursing, 6*(1), 43-51.

Apgar, V. (1953). Proposal for mew method of evaluation of newborn infant. *Anesthesia and Analgesia, 32,* 260-267.

Askin, D.F. (1995). Bacterial and fungal infections in the neonate. *Journal of Obstetric, Gynecologic, and Neonatal Nursing, 24*(7), 635-643.

Association of Women's Health, Obstetric and Neonatal Nurses. (1996). *Clinical Commentary: Perinatal group B streptococcal disease.* Washington, DC: Author.

Attico, N.B., Meyer, D.J., Bodin, H.J., & Dickman, D.S. (1990). Gestational age assessment. *American Family Physician, 41*(2), 553-560.

Auvenshine, M.A., & Enriquez, M.G. (1990). *Comprehensive Maternity Nursing: Perinatal and Women's Health.* Boston: Jones & Bartlett.

Babson, S.G., Behrman, R.E., & Lessel, R. (1970). Liveborn birthweights for gestational age of white middle class infants. *Pediatrics, 45, 937-944.*

Baird, P.B. & Witt, C.L. (1996). Neonatal glucose screening. *Neonatal Network 15*(7), 63-66.

Bakht, F.R., & Gentry, L.O. (1992). Toxoplasmosis in pregnancy: An emerging concern for family physicians. *American Family Physician, 45(4),* 1683-1689.

Ballard, J.L., Khoury, J.C., Wedig, K., Wang, L., Ellers-Walsman, B.L., & Lipp, R. (1991). New Ballard score, expanded to include extremely premature infants. *Journal of Pediatrics, 119*(3), 417-423.

Ballard, J.L., Novak, K.K., & Driver, M.A. (1979). A simplified score for assessment of fetal maturation of newly born infants. *Journal of Pediatrics, 95*(6), 769-774.

Battaglia, F.C., & Lubchenco, L.O. (1967). A practical classification of newborn infants by weight and gestational age. *Journal of Pediatrics, 71,* 159-163.

Blackburn, S.T. (1990). Assessment of risk in the newborn: Neonatal growth and maturity. White Plains, NY: March of Dimes Birth Defects Foundation.

Blackburn, S.T. (1995). Hyperbilirubinemia and neonatal jaundice. *Neonatal Network, 14*(7), 15-25.

Blackburn, S.T. (1992). Vitamin K and hemorrhagic diseases of the newborn. In *Maternal, fetal and neonatal physiology: A clinical perspective.* Philadelphia: W.B. Saunders, 188-189.

Blackburn, S.T., & Loper, D.L. (1992). Thermoregulation. In *Maternal, fetal, and neonatal physiology: A clinical perspective.* Philadelphia: W.B. Saunders, 677-697.

Bland, R.D. (1992). Formation of fetal lung liquid and its removal near birth. In R.A. Polin & W.W. Fox (Eds.), *Fetal and neonatal physiology.* Philadelphia: W.B. Saunders.

Bliss-Holtz, J. (1989). Comparison of rectal, axillary, and inguinal temperatures in full-term newborn infants. *Nursing Research, 38*(2), 85-87.

Bliss-Holtz, J. (1991). Determining cold-stress in full-term newborn through temperature site comparisons. *Scholarly Inquiry for Nursing Practice: An International Journal, 5,* 113-123.

Bliss-Holtz, J. (1993). Determination of thermoregulatory state in full-term infants. *Nursing Research,* 204-207.

Bliss-Holtz, J. (1995). Methods of newborn infant temperature monitoring: A research review. *Issues in Comprehensive Pediatric Nursing, 18,* 287-298.

Bloom, R.S., Cropley, C., & AHA/AAP Neonatal Resuscitation Program Steering Committee. (1995). *Textbook of neonatal resuscitation.* Chicago: American Academy of Pediatrics.

Brazelton, T.B. (1984). *Neonatal behavioral assessment scale* (2nd ed.). Spastics International Medical Publications, in association with London: William Heinemann Medical Books Ltd. & Philadelphia: J.B. Lippincott.

Brown, A.L., Fernhoff, P.M., Milner, J., McEwen, C., & Elsas, L.J. (1981). Racial differences in the incidence of congenital hypothyroidism. *Journal of Pediatrics, 99,* 934-936.

Brown, L.P. (1992). Breastfeeding and jaundice: Cause of concerns? *NAACOG's Clinical Issues, 3*(4), 613-19.

Brown, Z., Benedetti, J., Ashley, R., Burchett, S., Selkey, S., Berry, S., Vontver, L., & Corey, L. (1992). Neonatal herpes simplex virus infection in relation to asymptomatic maternal infection at the time of labor. *The New England Journal of Medicine, 324,* 1247-52.

Bruck, K. (1978). Non-shivering thermogenesis and brown adipose tissue in relation to age, and their integration in the thermoregulatory system. In O. Lindberg (Ed.), *Brown adipose tissue.* New York: Elsevier, 117-154.

Brueggemeyer, A. (1993). Neonatal thermoregulation. In C. Kenner & A. Brueggemeyer (Eds.), *Comprehensive neonatal nursing: A physiologic perspective.* Philadelphia: W.B. Saunders, 247-262.

Bullock, B. (1992). Pathophysiology, adaptations and alterations in function. In J. Whatley, et. al., *Biophysical development of children.* Philadelphia: J.B. Lippincott Company.

Buzby, M. (1991). Assessment of hyperbilirubinemia in full term infants: Part II. *Journal of Pediatric Health Care,* 210-212.

Carmack, M.A., & Prober, C.G. (1993). Neonatal herpes: Vexing dilemmas and reasons for hope. *Current Opinion in Pediatrics, 5,* 21-8.

Carter, B., Haverkamp, A., & Merenstein, G. (1993). The definition of acute perinatal asphyxia. *Clinics in Perinatology, 20,* 287-304.

Cavaliere, T.A. (1995). Pharmacologic treatment of neonatal sepsis: Antimicrobial agents and immunotherapy. *Journal of Obstetric, Gynecologic, and Neonatal Nursing, 24*(7), 647-58.

Centers for Disease Control and Prevention. (1988). Prevention of perinatal transmission of hepatitis B virus: Prenatal screening of all pregnant women for hepatitis B surface antigen. *Mortality and Morbidity Weekly Report, 37,* 341-346.

Centers for Disease Control and Prevention. (1991). Hepatitis B virus: A comprehensive strategy for eliminating hepatitis B transmission in the United States through universal childhood vaccination. *Mortality and Morbidity Weekly Report, 40,* 1-25.

REFERENCES

Centers for Disease Control and Prevention. (1993). Recommendations for the prevention and management of chlamydia trachomatis infections. *Mortality and Morbidity Weekly Report, 42*, 1-39.

Centers for Disease Control and Prevention. (1994). *HIV/AIDS Surveillance Report* (1st semi-annual ed.), *6*(1), 1-15.

Centers for Disease Control and Prevention. (1996). Prevention of perinatal group B streptococcal disease: A public health prospective. *Morbidity and Mortality Weekly Report, 45*, 1-24.

Christensen, R.D., & Rothstein, G. (1979). Pitfalls in the interpretation of leukocyte counts of newborn infants. *American Journal of Clinical Pathology, 72*, 608-611.

Clark, F.I., & James, E.J.P. (1995). Twenty-seven years of experience with oral vitamin K_1 therapy in neonates. *Journal of Pediatrics, 127*(2), 301-304.

Cloherty, J.P. (1991). Neonatal hyperbilirubinemia. In J.P. Cloherty & A.R. Stark (Eds.). *Manual of neonatal care*, (3rd ed.). Boston: Little Brown, 298-334.

Cole, M.D. (1991). New factors associated with the incidence of hypoglycemia: A research study. *Neonatal Network, 10*(4), 47-50.

Coles, E.C., & Valman, H.B. (1979). Hats for the newborn infant (letter). *British Medical Journal, 2*(6192), 734-735.

Copper, R., & Goldenberg, R. (1990). Catecholamine secretion in fetal adaptation to stress. *Journal of Obstetric, Gynecologic, & Neonatal Nursing, 19*, 223-226.

Cornblath, M., & Schwartz, R. (1993). Hypoglycemia in the neonate. *Journal of Pediatric Endocrinology, 6*(2), 113-129.

Cornblath, M., Schwartz, R., Aynsley-Green, A., & Lloyd, J.K. (1990). Hypoglycemia in infancy: The need for a rational definition. A CIBA Foundation discussion meeting. *Pediatrics, 85,*(5), 834-837.

Cowett, R. (1992). Hypoglycemia and hyperglycemia in the newborn. In R.A. Polin & W.W. Fox (Eds.), *Fetal and neonatal physiology.* Philadelphia: W.B. Saunders.

Crane, M.J. (1992). Clinical update: The diagnosis and management of maternal and congenital syphilis. *Journal of Nurse-Midwifery, 37*(1), 4-15.

Crockett, M. (1995). Physiology of the neonatal immune system. *Journal of Obstetric, Gynecologic, and Neonatal Nursing, 24*, 627-634.

D'Apolito, K. (1994). Hats used to maintain body temperature. *Neonatal Network, 13*(5), 93-94.

Darnall, R.A. (1987). The thermophysiology of the newborn infant. *Medical Instrumentation (1)*, 16-22.

Desmond, M.M., Franklin, R.R., Valbona, C., Hill, R.M., Plumb, R., Arnold, H., & Watts, J. (1963). The clinical behavior of the newly born: 1. The term baby. *The Journal of Pediatrics, 62*, 307-325.

Dodd, V. (1996). Gestational age assessment. *Neonatal Network, 15*(1), 27-36.

Dodman, N. (1987). Newborn temperature control. *Neonatal Network, 5*(6), 19-23.

Downey, J.C., & Cloherty, J.P. (1991). Metabolic problems. In J.P. Cloherty & A.R. Starks (Eds.), *Manual of neonatal care.* (3rd ed.) Boston: Little Brown, 431-437.

Dubowitz, L.M.S., Dubowitz, V., & Goldberg, C. (1970). Clinical assessment of gestational age in the newborn infant. *Journal of Pediatrics, 77*(1), 1-10.

Eichenwald, E.C. (1991). Meconium aspiration. In J.P. Cloherty & A.R. Stark (Eds.), *Manual of neonatal care* (3rd ed.). Boston: Little Brown, 246-250.

Falconer, A.D., & Lake, D.M. (1982). Circumstances influencing umbilical-cord plasma catecholamines at delivery. *British Journal of Obstetrics and Gynecology, 9*, 44-49.

Felblinger, D.M., & Weitkamp, T.L. (1993). In C. Kenner et al. (Eds.), *Comprehensive neonatal nursing care: A physiologic perspective.* Philadelphia: W.B. Saunders, 215-230.

Fowler, K.B., Stagno, S., & Pass, R.F. (1993). Maternal age and congenital cytomegalovirus infection: Screening of two diverse newborn populations, 1980-1990. *Journal of Infectious Diseases, 168*, 552-556.

Freitag-Koontz, M.J. (1996). Prevention of hepatitis B and C: Transmission during pregnancy and the first year of life. *Journal of Perinatal and Neonatal Nursing, 10(2)*, 40-55.

Gartner, L.M., & Lee, K.S. (1992). Unconjugated hyperbili-rubinemia. In A. Fanaroff & R. Martin (Eds.), *Neonatal-perinatal medicine: Diseases of the fetus and infant* (5th ed.). St. Louis: Mosby-Year Book, 1075-1103.

Girard, J., & Narkewicz, M. (1992). Role of glucoregulatory hormones on hepatic glucose metabolism during the perinatal period. In R.A. Polin & W.W. Fox (Eds.), *Fetal and neonatal physiology.* Philadelphia: W. B. Saunders, 390-405.

Glatzl-Hawlik, M.A., & Bell, E. (1992). Environmental temperature control. In R.A. Polin & W.W. Fox (Eds.), *Fetal and neonatal physiology.* Philadelphia: W. B. Saunders, 515-526.

Golding, J., Greenwood, R., Birmingham, K., & Mott, M. (1992). Childhood cancer, intramuscular vitamin K, and pethidine given during labour. *British Medical Journal, 305*, 341-346.

Goldsmith, J.P., & Starrett, A.L. (1991). The neonatal effects of anesthetic agents and techniques. In J.H. Diaz (Ed.), *Perinatal anesthesia and critical care.* Philadelphia: W.B. Saunders.

Gomella, T.L. (1992). *Hyperglycemia in neonatology: Management, procedures, on-call problems, diseases, drugs.* Norwalk, CT: Appleton & Lange, 210-213.

Gourley, G. R. (1992). Pathophysiology of breastmilk jaundice. In R.A. Polin & W.W. Fox (Eds.), *Fetal and neonatal physiology.* Philadelphia: W.B. Saunders, 1173-1179.

Assessment of Risk in the Term Newborn

Please remove and complete the evaluation, fold and staple it to reveal the postage-paid portion, and post it in a U.S. mailbox. (Note: Independent study takers can submit the evaluation with their tests and fees for grading; group study participants can give the evaluation to their facilitator.) Thank you in advance for your time. Your responses are important to us as we plan additional continuing education activities.

1. **State(s) in which you currently practice**

   _____

2. **Professional identification** *(Check all that apply.)*
   ☐ Registered nurse
   ☐ Nurse practitioner
   ☐ Clinical nurse specialist
   ☐ Certified nurse-midwife
   ☐ Childbirth educator
   ☐ Nursing student
   ☐ Other *(Please identify.)* _____

3. **Educational degree(s)** *(Check all that apply.)*
   ☐ Diploma nurse
   ☐ Associate degree
   ☐ Baccalaureate in nursing
   ☐ Baccalaureate in other field *(Please identify.)*
   _____

   ☐ Master's in nursing
   ☐ Master's in other field *(Please identify.)*
   _____

   ☐ Doctorate in nursing
   ☐ Doctorate in other field *(Please identify.)*
   _____

4. **Area(s) of certification**

   _____

5. **Current employment setting**
   ☐ Hospital
   ☐ Clinic
   ☐ Private practice
   ☐ Other *(Please identify.)* _____

6. **Type of work**
   ☐ Administration
   ☐ Education—academic/clinical
   ☐ Clinical practice
   ☐ Public health
   ☐ Other *(Please identify.)* _____

7. **Length of time employed in the health care field**
   ☐ <1 year
   ☐ 1 to 2 years
   ☐ 2 to 10 years
   ☐ 10 to 20 years
   ☐ >20 years

8. **How did you find out about this module?**
   ☐ March of Dimes (MOD) chapter
   ☐ MOD national office
   ☐ MOD website
   ☐ Conference
   ☐ Place of employment
   ☐ Peer/Colleague recommendation
   ☐ Other *(Please identify.)* _____
   _____

9. **Have you used other MOD nursing modules?**
   ☐ Yes   ☐ No   ☐ Unsure

10. **If you are a prior module user, how many modules have you used?** _____

11. **If you are a prior module user, when was the last time you used a module?**
    ☐ <1 month ago
    ☐ 1 month to 1 year ago
    ☐ 1 to 2 years ago
    ☐ >2 years ago

12. **How did you use this module?**
    ☐ Independent study for continuing education credit
    ☐ Group study for continuing education credit
    ☐ As a learning tool without continuing education credit
    ☐ Other *(Please identify.)* _____
    _____

13. **Time required to read the module and complete the independent study test, if applicable**
    _____hours   _____minutes   ☐ Not applicable

14. **Time required to read the module and participate in the facilitated group study, if applicable**
    _____hours   _____minutes   ☐ Not applicable

Rate each of the following:

	Excellent	Very Good	Good	Fair	Poor	N/A
15. Cognitive objectives	_____	_____	_____	_____	_____	_____
16. Relationship of cognitive objectives to the overall purpose of the module	_____	_____	_____	_____	_____	_____
17. Expected practice outcomes	_____	_____	_____	_____	_____	_____
18. Key concepts	_____	_____	_____	_____	_____	_____
19. Content	_____	_____	_____	_____	_____	_____
20. Clinical application	_____	_____	_____	_____	_____	_____
21. Group discussion items	_____	_____	_____	_____	_____	_____
22. References	_____	_____	_____	_____	_____	_____
23. Supplementary materials	_____	_____	_____	_____	_____	_____
24. Overall quality of the module	_____	_____	_____	_____	_____	_____
25. Effectiveness of the module as teaching/learning material	_____	_____	_____	_____	_____	_____
26. Effectiveness of module as a means to increase awareness of the issue/topic	_____	_____	_____	_____	_____	_____

(Continued on other side)

27. Which may change as a result of completing this module?
- ☐ Your attitude
- ☐ Your knowledge base
- ☐ Your skill level
- ☐ Other *(Please identify.)* _____

28. How might your use of the nursing process be affected by the module?
- ☐ Improved data collection
- ☐ Improved client assessment
- ☐ Improved accuracy in nursing diagnoses
- ☐ Improved discharge planning
- ☐ Improved (more appropriate) nursing interventions
- ☐ Improved evaluation of nursing care
- ☐ Other *(Please identify.)* _____

29. Would you recommend this module to a colleague?
- ☐ Yes   ☐ No   ☐ Unsure

30. How can the module be improved?
_____
_____
_____

31. Suggestions for future module topics
_____
_____
_____

32. Other comments
_____
_____
_____

← Fold Line

BUSINESS REPLY MAIL
FIRST CLASS • PERMIT NO. 2000 • WHITE PLAINS, NY

POSTAGE WILL BE PAID BY ADDRESSEE

March of Dimes Birth Defects Foundation
Education Services
1275 Mamaroneck Avenue
White Plains, NY 10602-9989

NO POSTAGE
NECESSARY IF
MAILED
IN THE
UNITED STATES

Fold Line →

FOR FACILITATORS ONLY

1. Number of participants attending the study
_____

2. Location of the study
_____

3. Date of the study
_____

4. Length time for the study
_____

5. When was the study held?
- ☐ During compensated on-duty time
- ☐ As an overtime (paid) activity
- ☐ On noncompensated time
- ☐ Other *(Please identify.)* _____

6. Reasons for the group study *(Check all that apply.)*
- ☐ To offer/obtain continuing education credit
- ☐ To cross-train staff
- ☐ To enhance clinical skills
- ☐ Other *(Please identify.)* _____
_____

7. Did you offer/obtain continuing education credit for the module from the March of Dimes?
- ☐ Yes   ☐ No

8. How could the group study process be improved?
_____
_____

REFERENCES

Grant, A. (1996). Varicella infection and toxoplasmosis in pregnancy. *The Journal of Perinatal and Neonatal Nursing, 10*(2), 17-29.

Greer, F. (1995). Vitamin K deficiency and hemorrhage in infancy. *Clinics in Perinatology, 22*, 759-767.

Greer, P.S. (1988). Head coverings for the newborns under radiant warmers. *Journal of Obstetric, Gynecologic and Neonatal Nursing*, July-August, 265-271.

Guerina, N.G. (1991). Bacterial and fungal infections. In J.P. Cloherty & A.R. Stark (Eds.), *Manual of neonatal care* (3rd ed.). Boston: Little, Brown, & Company.

Gunderson, L.M., & Gumm, B. (1992). Neonatal acquired immunodeficiency syndrome: Human immunodeficiency virus infection and acquired immunodeficiency syndrome in the infant. In C. Kenner et al. (Eds.), *Comprehensive neonatal nursing care: A physiologic perspective*. Philadelphia: W.B. Saunders, 940-967.

Gunderson, L.P., Cantu, D., Vaello, L.R., & Brueggemeyer, A.E. (1993). Care of high-risk infants and their families. In C.A. Kenner & A. MacLaren (Eds.), *Essentials of maternal and neonatal nursing*. Springhouse PA: Springhouse Corporation, 422-487.

Guthrie, R., & Susi, A. (1963). A simple phenylalanine method for detecting phenylketonuria in large populations of newborn infants. *Pediatrics, 32*, 338-343.

Haddock, B., Vincent, P., & Merrow, D. (1986). Axillary and rectal temperatures of full-term neonates: Are they different? *Neonatal Network, 5*(1), 36-40.

Hall, S.M. (1992). Congenital toxoplasmosis. *British Medical Journal, 305*, 291-297.

Hallam, A., & Kerlin, P. (1991). Viral hepatitis A to E. *Australian Family Physician, 20*, 762-3, 766-770.

Hammerschlag, M.R. (1994). Chlamydia trachomatis in children. *Pediatric Annals, 23*(7), 349-353.

Hanold, K.C., Kemp, V.H., & Nelms, T.P. (1993). In C.A. Kenner & A. MacLaren (Eds.), *Essentials of maternal and neonatal nursing*. Springhouse, PA: Springhouse, 220.

Hanson, C.A. (1994). Peripheral blood and bone marrow: Morphology, counts and differentials, and reactive disorders. In K.D. McClatchey (Ed.), *Clinical Laboratory Medicine*. Baltimore: Williams & Wilkins, 827-865.

Hasan, R., Inoue, S., & Banerjee, A. (1993). Higher white blood cell counts and band forms in newborns delivered vaginally compared with those delivered by cesarean section. *American Journal of Clinical Pathology, 100*, 116-118.

Hawdon, J.M., & Ward, M.P. (1993). Metabolic adaptation in small for gestational age infants. *Archives of Diseases in Children, 68*, 262-268.

Hawdon, J.M., Platt-Ward, M.P., & Aynsley-Green, A. (1992). Patterns of metabolic adaptation for preterm and term neonates in the first postnatal week. *Archives of Diseases in Children, 67*, 357-365.

Haywood, J., Coghill, C., Carlo, W., & Ross, M. (1993). Assessment and management of respiratory dysfunction. In C. Kenner, A. Brueggemeyer, & L.P. Gunderson (Eds.), *Comprehensive neonatal nursing: A physiologic perspective*. Philadelphia: W.B. Saunders, 294-335.

Hicks, B.A., & Altman, R.P. (1993). The jaundiced newborn. *Pediatric Clinics of North America, 40*(6), 1161-75.

Hill, A. (1992). Development of tone and reflexes in fetus and newborn. In R.A. Polin & W.W. Fox (Eds.), *Fetal and neonatal physiology*. Philadelphia: W.B. Saunders, 1578-1587.

Holditch-Davis, D. (1993). Neonatal sleep-wake states. In Kenner et al. (Eds.), *Comprehensive neonatal nursing care: A physiologic perspective*. Philadelphia: W.B. Saunders, 940-967.

Hughes, S.C., & DeVore, J.S. (1993). Psychologic and alternative techniques for obstetric anesthesia. In S.M. Shnider & G. Levinson (Eds.), *Anesthesia for obstetrics* (3rd ed.). Philadelphia: Williams and Wilkins.

Hunter, L.P. (1991). Measurement of axillary temperatures in neonates. *Western Journal of Nursing Research, 13*, 324-335.

Ingram, D.L. (1994). Neisseria gonorrhoeae in children. *Pediatric Annals, 23*(7), 341-345.

Irons, M. (1993). Screening for metabolic disorders: How are we doing? *Pediatric Clinics of North America, 40*(5), 1073-1085.

Jones, B.M. (1990). A physiologic approach to identifying neonates at risk for kernicterus. *Journal of Obstetric, Gynecologic, and Neonatal Nursing*, 313-318.

Judson, F.N., & Ehret, J. (1994). Laboratory diagnosis of sexually transmitted infections. *Pediatric Annals, 23*(7), 361-369.

Kalhan, S. (1993). Metabolism of glucose and methods of investigation in the fetus and newborn. In R.A. Polin & W.W. Fox (Eds.), *Fetal and neonatal physiology*. Philadelphia: W.B. Saunders, 357-372.

Kaminski, J., & Hall, W. (1996). The effect of soothing music on neonatal behavioral states in the hospital newborn nursery. *Neonatal Network, 15*(1), 45-54.

Karp, T., Scardino, C., & Butler, L. (1995) Glucose metabolism in the neonate: The short and sweet of it. *Neonatal Network, 14*(8), 17-23.

Kenner, C., Brueggemeyer, A., & Gunderson, L.P. (1993). *Comprehensive neonatal nursing*. Philadelphia: W.B. Saunders.

Kirsten, D. (1996). Patent ductus arteriosus in the preterm infant. *Neonatal Network, 15*(2), 19-26.

Kisker, C.T. (1992). Pathophysiology of bleeding disorders in the newborn. In R.A. Polin & W.W. Fox (Eds.), *Fetal and neonatal physiology*. Philadelphia: W.B. Saunders, 1384-1386.

Klaus, M.H., & Fanaroff, A. (1993). *Care of the high-risk neonate.* (4th ed.). Philadelphia: W.B. Saunders.

Kleigman, R.M. (1993). Problems in metabolic adaptation: Glucose, calcium, and magnesium. In M.H. Klaus & A.A. Fanaroff (Eds.), *Care of the high-risk neonate* (4th ed.). Philadelphia: W.B. Saunders, 282-290.

Klein, J.O., & Marcy, S.M. (1995). Bacterial sepsis and meningitis. In J.S. Remington & J.O.Klein (Eds.), *Infectious diseases of the fetus and newborn* (4th ed.). Philadelphia: W.B. Saunders, 835-890.

Kunnel, M.T., O'Brien, C., Munro, B.H., & Medoff-Cooper, B. (1988). Comparisons of rectal, femoral, axillary, and skin-to-mattress temperatures in stable neonates. *Nursing Research, 37,* 162-164, 189.

Ladewig, P., London, M., & Olds, S. (1994). *Essentials of maternal-newborn nursing* (3rd ed.). Redwood City, California: Addison-Wesley Nursing.

Le Blanc, M.H. (1992). Neonatal heat transfer. In R.A. Polin and W.W. Fox (Eds.), *Fetal and neonatal physiology.* Philadelphia: W.B. Saunders, 483-488.

Letko, M. (1996). Understanding the Apgar Score. *Journal of Obstetric, Gynecologic, & Neonatal Nursing, 25,* 299-303.

Leuthner, S.R., Jansen, R.D., & Hageman, J.R. (1994). Cardiopulmonary resuscitation of the newborn: An update. *Pediatric Clinics of North America, 41*(5), 893-907.

Lewis, D.B., & Wilson, C.B. (1992). Host defense mechanisms against bacteria, fungi, viruses, and nonviral intracellular pathogens. In R. Polin & W. Fox (Eds.), *Fetal and neonatal physiology.* Philadelphia: W.B. Saunders, 1404-1427.

Lin, H.C., et. al. (1989). Accuracy and reliability of glucose reflectance meters in the high-risk neonate. *Journal of Pediatrics, 115,* 998.

Lott, J.W. (1993). *Neonatal infection: Assessment, diagnosis, and management.* Petaluma, CA: NICU Ink, 23-35.

Lott, J.W., & Kenner, C. (1994a). Keeping up with neonatal infections: Designer bugs, part I. *MCN: The Journal of Maternal-Child Nursing, 19,* 207-213.

Lott, J.W., & Kenner, C. (1994b). Keeping up with neonatal infections: Designer bugs, part II. *MCN: The Journal of Maternal-Child Nursing, 19,* 264-271.

Lott, J.W., Nelson, K., Fahrner, R., & Kenner, C. (1993). Assessment and management of immunologic dysfunction. In C. Kenner, A. Brueggemeyer, & L.P. Gunderson, (Eds.), *Comprehensive neonatal nursing: A physiologic perspective.* Philadelphia: W.B. Saunders, 553-581.

Lubchenco, L.O., Searles, D.T., & Brazie, J.V. (1972). Neonatal mortality rate: Relationship to birthweight and gestational age. *Journal of Pediatrics, 81,* 814-822.

Lumb, T.M. (1994). Group B streptococcus revisited. *Pediatric Nursing, 20*(6), 578-80.

Mahlmeister, L. (1996). Perinatal group B streptococcal infections: The nurse's role in identification and prophylaxis. *Journal of Perinatal and Neonatal Nursing, 10*(2), 1-16.

Maisels, M.J. (1994). Jaundice. In G.B. Avery., M.A. Fletcher & M.G. MacDonald (Eds.), *Neonatology: Pathophysiology and management of the newborn,* (4th ed.). Philadelphia: J.B. Lippincott, 630-725.

Maisels, M.J., Gifford, K., Antle, C.E., & Leib, G.R. (1988). Jaundice in the healthy newborn infant: A new approach to an old problem. *Pediatrics, 81*(4), 505-511.

Mayfield, S.R., Bhatia, J., Nakamura, K.T., Rios, G.R., & Bell, E.F. (1984). Temperature measurement in term and preterm neonates. *The Journal of Pediatrics, 104,* 271-275.

McFadden, E.A. (1991). The wallaby phototherapy system: A new approach to phototherapy. *Journal of Pediatric Nursing, 6*(3), 206-208.

McGowan, J., Hagedorn, M., & Hay, W. (1993). Glucose homeostasis. In G.B. Merenstein & S.L. Gardner (Eds.), *Handbook of neonatal intensive care* (3rd ed.). St. Louis: Mosby, 169-183.

Mehta, A., Wōolton, R., Cheng, K.L., Penfold, P., Halliday, D., & Stacey, T.E. (1987). Effect of diazoxide or glucagon on hepatic glucose production rate during extreme hypoglycemia. *Archive of Diseases in Children, 62,* 924-930.

Merenstein, G.B., & Gardner, S.L. (1993). *Handbook of neonatal intensive care* (3rd ed.). St. Louis: Mosby.

Miles, S.A., Balden, E., Magpantay, L., Wei, L., Leiblein, A., Hofheinz, D., Toedter, G., Stiehm, E.R., Bryson, Y., & The Southern California Pediatric AIDS Consortium. (1993). Rapid serologic testing with immune-complex-dissociated HIV p24 antigen for early detection of HIV infection in neonates. *The New England Journal of Medicine, 328,* 297-302.

Moslet, V., & Hansen, E.S. (1992). A review of vitamin K, epilepsy and pregnancy. *Acta Neurol Scand, 85,* 39-43.

Nash, P. (1996). Common neonatal complications. In K.R. Simpson & P.A. Creehan (Eds.), *AWHONN'S perinatal nursing.* Philadelphia: Lippincott-Raven, 355-375.

Nelson, K., & Emery, E.S. (1993). Birth asphyxia and the neonatal brain: What do we know and when do we know it? *Clinics in Perinatology, 20,* 327-344.

Newman, T., & Maisels, M.J. (1992). Evaluation and treatment of jaundice in the term newborn: A kinder, gentler approach. *Pediatrics, 89*(5), 809-823.

Oski, F.A. (1993). The erythrocyte and its disorders. In D.G. Nathan & F.A. Oski (Eds.), *Hematology of infancy and childhood* (4th ed., Vol. 1). Philadelphia: W.B. Saunders, 18-43.

Padbury, J.F., & Ogata, E.S. (1992). Glucose metabolism during the transition to postnatal life. In R.A. Polin & W.W. Fox (Eds.), *Fetal and neonatal physiology.* Philadelphia: W.B. Saunders, 402-405.

REFERENCES

Pildes, R.S., & Lilian, L.D. (1992). Metabolic and endocrine disorders. In A.A. Faranoff & J.M. Martin, (Eds.), *Neonatal-perinatal medicine: Diseases of the fetus and infant* (5th ed.). St Louis: Mosby-Year Book, 1152-1292.

Polinski, C. (1996). The value of the white blood cell count and differential in the prediction of neonatal sepsis. *Neonatal Network, 7,* 13-23.

Remington, J.S., & Klein, J.O. (1995). *Infectious diseases of the fetus and newborn infant* (4th ed.). Philadelphia: W.B. Saunders.

Remington, J.S., McLeod, R., & Desmonts, G. (1995). Toxoplasmosis. In J.S. Remington & J.O. Klein (Eds.), *Infectious diseases of the fetus and newborn infant* (4th ed.). Philadelphia: W.B. Saunders, 140-267.

Rosenfeld, E.A., Hageman, J.R., & Yogev, R. (1993). Tuberculosis in infancy in the 1990s. *Pediatric Clinics of North America, 40,* 1087-1103.

Rowe, M.I., Weinberg, G., & Andrews, W. (1983). Reduction of neonatal heat loss by an insulated head cover. *Journal of Pediatric Surgery, 18*(6), 909-913.

Ruchala, P., Seibold, L., & Stremsterfer, K. (1996). Validating assessment of neonatal jaundice with transcutaneous bilirubin measurement. *Neonatal Network, 15*(4), 33-37.

Schuchat, A., & Wenger, J.D. (1994). Epidemiology of group B streptococcal disease. *Epidemiology Review, 16,* 374-401.

Shannon, L. (1995). Clinical perspectives and current trends of HIV infection in the newborn and child. *Neonatal Network, 14*(3), 21-34.

Shaw, N. (1993). Assessment and management of hematologic dysfunction. In C. Kenner, et al. (Eds.), *Comprehensive neonatal nursing: A physiologic perspective.* Philadelphia: W.B. Saunders, 582-634.

Sinclair, J. (1976). Metabolic rate and temperature control. In C.A. Smith & N.N. Nelson (Eds.), *The physiology of the newborn infant* (4th ed.). Springfield, IL: Charles C. Thomas.

Smith, M., & Teele, D. (1995). Tuberculosis. In J.S. Remington & J.O. Klein (Eds.), *Infectious diseases of the fetus and newborn* (4th ed.). Philadelphia: W.B. Saunders, 1074-1086.

Snapp, B., (1996). Hemorrhagic disease of the newborn and vitamin K. *Mother Baby Journal, 1*(4), 17-23.

Sparks, J.W., & Cetin, I. (1992). Intrauterine growth and nutrition. In R.A. Polin and W.W. Fox (Eds.), *Fetal and neonatal physiology.* Philadelphia: W.B. Saunders, 179-197.

Stagno, S. (1995). Cytomegalovirus. In J.S. Remington & J.O.Klein (Eds.), *Infectious diseases of the fetus and newborn* (4th ed.). Philadelphia: W.B. Saunders, 312-353.

Starling, S.P. (1994). Syphilis in infants and young children. *Pediatric Annals, 23*(7), 334-340.

Stephen, S.B., & Sexton, P.R. (1987). Neonatal axillary temperatures: Increases in readings over time. *Neonatal Network, 5*(6), 25-28.

Stiles, A.D., & Cloherty, J.P. (1991). Metabolic problems. In J.P. Cloherty & A. R. Stark, (Eds.), *Manual of neonatal care* (3rd ed.). Boston: Little, Brown & Company, 339-343.

Stokowski, L.C. (1992). Metabolic disorders. In P. Beachy & J. Deacon (Eds.), *Core curriculum for neonatal intensive care nursing.* Philadelphia: W.B. Saunders, 281-286.

Stothers, J.K. (1981). Head insulation and heat loss in the newborn. *Archives of Disease in Childhood, 56,* 530-534.

Strodtbeck, F. (1995). Viral infections of the newborn. *Journal of Obstetric, Gynecologic, and Neonatal Nursing, 24*(7), 659-667.

TePas, K.E. (1988). *Thermoregulation in newborns.* White Plains: March of Dimes Birth Defects Foundation.

Thoman, E.B. (1990). Sleeping and waking states in infancy: A functional perspective. *Neuroscience and Biobehavioral Reviews, 14,* 93-107.

Thomas, K. (1994). Thermoregulation in neonates. *Neonatal Network, 13*(2), 15-22.

Tilman, J. (1992). Syphilis: An old disease, a contemporary perinatal problem. *Journal of Obstetric, Gynecologic, and Neonatal Nursing, 21*(3), 209-213.

Trotter, C.W. (1993). Gestational age assessment. In E.P. Tappero & M.E. Honeyfield (Eds.), *Physical assessment of the newborn: A comprehensive approach to the art of physical examination.* Petaluma, CA: NICU Ink.

Tulchinsky, T.H., Patton, M.M., Randolph, L.A., Meyer, M.R., & Linden, J.V. (1993). Mandating vitamin K prophylaxis for newborns in New York state. *American Journal of Public Health, 83*(8), 1166-1168.

Urang, S. (1990). Cytomegalovirus infection in pregnancy. *Journal of Nurse-Midwifery, 35*(5), 299-306.

Usta, I., Mercer, B.M., & Sibai, B.M. (1995). Risk factors for meconium aspiration syndrome. *Obstetrics & Gynecology, 86*(2), 230-234.

Volpe, J.J. (1987). Hypoxic-ischemic encephalopathy: Clinical aspects. In *Neurology of the newborn* (2nd ed.). Philadelphia: W.B. Saunders.

Weiss, M. (1991). Tympanic infrared thermometry in full-term and preterm neonates. *Clinical Pediatrics, 30*(4), 42-45.

Weiss, M., Poeltler, D., & Gocka, I. (1994). Infrared tympanic thermometry for neonatal temperature assessment. *Journal of Gynecologic, Obstetric, and Neonatal Nursing, 23,* 798-804.

Werner, E.J. (1995). Neonatal polycythemia and hyperviscosity. *Clinics in Perinatology, 22,* 693-710.

REFERENCES

Whatley, J.H., & Schlosser, S.P. (1992). Biophysical development of children. In B. Bullock & P. Rosendahl (Eds.), *Pathophysiology: Adaptations and alterations in function* (3rd ed.). Philadelphia: J.B. Lippincott Company.

Whitington, P.F., & Gartner, L.M. (1992). Disorder of bilirubin metabolism. In *Hematology of infancy and children.* Philadelphia: W.B. Saunders, 74.

Whitley, R.J. (1995). Herpes Simplex Virus Infections. In J.S. Remington & J.O.Klein (Eds.), *Infectious diseases of the fetus and newborn infant* (4th ed.). Philadelphia: W.B. Saunders.

Whitsett, J.A., Pryhuber, G.S., Rice, W.R., Werner, B.B., & Wert, S.E. (1994). Acute respiratory disorder, In G.B. Avery, M.A. Fletcher & M.G. MacDonald (Eds.), *Neonatology pathophysiology and management of the newborn* (4th ed.). Philadelphia: J.B. Lippincott, 429-451.

Williams, C.E., Mallard, C., Tan, W., & Gluckman, P. (1993). Pathophysiology of perinatal asphyxia. *Clinics in Perinatology, 20,* 305-325.

Witek-Janusek, L., & Cusak, C. (1994). Neonatal sepsis: Confronting the challenge. *Critical Care Nursing Clinics of North America, 6*(2), 405-419.

Witt, C. (1991). Neonatal consequences of asphyxia. *NAACOG's Clinical Issues, 2*(1), 48-77.

Wong, D. (1997). Health problems of the newborn. In D. Wong, (Ed.), *Whaley and Wong's essentials of pediatrics,* (5th ed.). St. Louis: Mosby-Year Book, 253-256.

Wright, L., Brown, A., & Davidson-Mundt, A. (1992). Newborn screening: The miracle and the challenge. *Journal of Pediatric Nursing, 7*(1), 26-42.

Yeh, T.F. (1991). *Neonatal therapeutics* (2nd ed.). St. Louis: Mosby-Year Book.

Yetman, R., Coody, D., West, M., Montgomery, D., & Brown, M. (1993). Comparison of temperature measurements by an aural infrared thermometer with measurements by traditional rectal and axillary techniques. *Journal of Pediatrics, 122,* 769-773.

Zeldis, J., & Crumpacher, C. (1995). Hepatitis. In J.S. Remington & J.O. Klein (Eds.), *Infectious diseases of the fetus and newborn infant* (3rd ed.). Phildadelphia: W.B. Saunders, 805-834.

33-805-97
ISBN 086525-074-X

March of Dimes
National Office
1275 Mamaroneck Avenue
White Plains, New York 10605
Telephone: (914) 428-7100
E-mail: profedu@modimes.org
Website: www.modimes.org